D1444542

Red Ribbons
Are Not Enough

Health Caregivers'
Stories About AIDS

Best regards —

Meredith Drench

Red Ribbons Are Not Enough

Health Caregivers' Stories About AIDS

Meredith E. Drench, PhD, PT

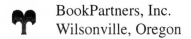

BookPartners, Inc.
Wilsonville, Oregon

Cover design by Richard Ferguson
Text design by Sheryl Mehary

BookPartners, Inc.
P.O. Box 922
Wilsonville, Oregon 97070

To my parents, Madeline and Daniel Drench, who have exemplified unconditional love, compassion, support, and wisdom.

To PJ Hurd, who personifies the word friend and whose belief in me, caring, encouragement, patience, and listening have been limitless.

To my dear friend and mentor, Ruthie Hall, who epitomizes what is real and good.

Acknowledgments

During the thousands of hours I gathered, reduced, analyzed, and synthesized data, I worked in solitude. *Red Ribbons,* in its new form, is based on a monograph I wrote in 1992, A Phenomenological Study of the Lived Experience of Health Care Professionals Working with People with Acquired Immune Deficiency Syndrome. Sharing my preparation of this manuscript with a cadre of scholarly and supportive individuals enhanced my experience and enjoyment. I particularly thank Sherry Penn, PhD, whose steadfast encouragement and friendship were unflagging.

I am indebted to the health care professionals who freely shared their insights, experiences, and time, allowing this study to come to fruition. Believing in this endeavor, they unabashedly told their stories to a "stranger," chronicling experiences which many of them had never before thought, articulated, or shared with another person. They are a very special group of compassionate individuals, and I thank them all.

I gratefully acknowledge and appreciate these fine people.

Table of Contents

Acknowledgments v

**Introduction—AIDS in Action: Challenges for
Health Care Professionals** 1
The Search for Answers Begins 4

**1   Understanding Acquired Immune Deficiency
Syndrome (AIDS)** 7
In the Beginning... 9
Compromises and Opportunities of the
Immune System. 12
Medical Illness or Social Disease. 15

2   Jessie: From Terminal to Chronic Illness 17
Sexual Preference and Work 18
Maintaining Emotional and Physical Health 20
Coming Up Through the Ranks 21
Finding that Little Speck — Challenges
of the Job 22
Twists to their Life Stories — Feeling
Overwhelmed 23
Experience is a Good Teacher 26
Feeling Effective, Feeling Gratified 27
Lip Service and Other Deeds — Feeling
Ineffective. 28
"Why Am I Doing This?" — Anger and
Frustration. 29
Carelessness and Needlesticks 30
Fear, Common Sense, and Transmission 32
The Uncertainty, the Unknown 33

I Was So Naive — What I've Learned 34
"Why Do You Do This?" 36
Innocence vs. Guilt 37
Staff Support Makes a Difference 38

3   Marlene: Endless Needs and Exhaustion 39
Giving Back 40
AIDS and Me — The Early Years 41
Making Choices. 42
Learning and Appreciating. 43
Drawing the Line. 47
A Small Part of a Big Tragedy 47
The Ties that Bind 48
My Challenges 49
My Family. 51
Risks and Fears 52
Fanning the Flames of Burnout 53
A Ship Came In, A Ship Went Out:
    Feeling Ineffective. 57
Feeling Effective, Being Effective 58
Maintaining Sanity and Other Helpful Thoughts . 60
The Media and Innocence vs. Guilt 61
Sexual Preference 63
The Privilege and the Challenge Continue 64

4   Elaine: Amidst the Frequency of Decline
        and Death. 67
Empowerment and Gratification 68
Sexual Preferences — The Patients' and
    My Own 69
Clinical and Other Challenges 70
Learning from The Emir 72
Shattering Illusions 74
Guilt, Innocence, and Avoidance 76
Fear and Comfort 78
Anxiety and Sorrow. 79

All-in-One: Most Effective, Least Effective 82
Team Support Keeps Me Going 83
Spirituality 84

5   Kim: Small Losses and Other Heartaches 87
On the Cutting Edge and Other Challenges 88
The Effectiveness–Ineffectiveness Continuum . . . 90
This Isn't the World I Made: Feeling Helpless . . . 92
Anger, Anger, Anger 93
Occasional Sadness, Occasional Laughter 95
Small Losses and Other Sorrows 96
Grilled Cheese Sandwiches and Saying
    Good-Bye 98
I'm Careful So I'm Not Afraid: The Security
    of Gloves 99
Coping with AIDS Work 100
Knowing Thyself 103

**6   Dennis: Separating the Disease from
    the People 105**
Making a Place for Myself 106
Challenges and Learning 107
Emotional Exhaustion and Endings 109
Making a Difference — Feeling Effective 112
Anger + Frustration = Ineffectiveness 113
Painful Professional Experiences Trigger
    Personal Responses 115
Coping is a Balancing Act 116

7   Steve: Identifying with the Patients 119
A Whole Realm of Feelings 120
Perspectives on Making a Difference 122
Surrounded by Illness — Lessons, Changes,
    and Burnout 124
Judgment, Education, and Caring 126

**8   Ann: Painfully Sad Watching Them
      Fade** **129**
"It's Never Too Late to Make a New Friend" —
      Sadness, Pain, and Loss. 130
Feeling Frustrated, Burned Out, and Ineffective. 132
"People Nobody Wants" — Choices,
      Challenges, and Excitement. 133
Living with a Chronic Disease. 136
Feeling Special — Advice for Other Health
      Professionals. 138

**9   Laura: Coping with the Progressive Nature
      of AIDS** **141**
Running and Valuing Life: Staying Balanced. . . 142
Entering the World of Children and AIDS 143
Looking at the Child as a Child, Not a Disease:
      Feeling Effective. 145
Evaluations, Not Treatments: Frustrations and
      Painful Experiences. 147
Fear, Anger, and Saving Lives 150
Funerals and Grief. 152
There are Limits: Lessons in Life 153
A Big Focus of My Life: AIDS and Me. 157

**10   Debbie: Vulnerability and the Meaning
      of Life.** **161**
Choices and Support 162
Intimate Moments 164
Sadness and Endings 165
A Veteran Amidst Turnover 167
On the Road to Burnout. 169
Life's Lessons on the AIDS Roller Coaster 171

**11 Mark: Discovering Value Judgments
and Biases** **175**
Accepting Patients After They've Been
Rejected by Others 176
Of Risks and Icebergs 180
Hostility and Secrets 182
Hard Lessons to Learn.................... 184

**12 Putting It All Together: What It's Like to
Work with People with AIDS** **189**
Riding the Roller Coaster: The Intensity of
Feelings......................... 190
Survival Skills: Dealing with the Meaning of
Loss and Death 195
All Learning Great and Small: Personal and
Professional Growth Issues 199
Changing Challenges of Care: Finding
Meaning in AIDS Care 201

13 Help and Hope........................ **205**
The Organized Approach............... 206
Shifting Winds...................... 208
The Chord of Change 209

Endnotes 211

About the Author....................... 217

Introduction

AIDS in Action: Challenges for Health Care Professionals

When I had a serious needlestick, I realized the practical reality of what I do. Despite all the counseling I give other people, I was an emotional wreck for a week.

Marlene, physician

Once upon a time, we had never heard of AIDS. Then, in the early 1980s we caught a tidbit from our televisions and newspapers about some mysterious virus. We got a little used to that. We heard about the Ebola Fever virus in a land far away and deer ticks spreading Lyme disease closer to home. Bacteria in hamburgers sickened, and even killed, some fast-food customers. Nevertheless, we believe that our scientists will no doubt find a cure for whatever ails us.

We began to hear more about this terrible scourge called GRID that seemed to spread like wildfire, but because it was Gay-Related Immune Deficiency, many people ignored the TV news and went back to eating dinner. We now know that GRID was a misnomer. This disease affects children and adults, whites and people of color, rich and poor, homosexuals and heterosexuals. The problem depresses immune systems so that people can't fight off certain bacteria, viruses, fungi, yeast, and protozoa. A new, accurate label was needed. GRID was renamed Acquired Immune Deficiency Syndrome — AIDS.

Once upon a time, AIDS was front-page news. Actor Rock Hudson died from it. Designer Perry Ellis died from it. Philosopher Michel Foucault died from it. Adolescent activist Ryan White died from it. We collectively gasped as our celebrities were cut down in their prime. The journey seemed to end in the same place — death. There was no cure.

Times have changed. There still is no cure, but there is good news. There's a longer time interval between the discovery of HIV-infection in a person and the diagnosis of full-blown AIDS. People with AIDS are treated earlier with more effective antiviral medication combinations. Better medications are available to treat opportunistic infections. There are many long-term survivors. Not everyone who is infected with the virus develops AIDS. People who were planning their wills and funerals are now returning to work. And yet, people still get sick, and people still die.

As the century draws to a close without a cure, the disease continues to rage worldwide. A certain apathy has set in. No longer a celebrity-sponsored disease, AIDS isn't front-page news anymore. It's old hat. Some people who had changed their high risk behaviors have become complacent and have resumed unsafe practices. Many people have put all their hope in the medicine cabinet of protease inhibitors, only to find that they don't help everyone or are too expensive to be accessible to all.

What's it like to be on the frontlines of a disease that is drifting out of our national consciousness? What's it like to help people cope with the terror of a devastating disease that can ravage the body and the soul? What's the impact on your marriage after you get stuck with a dirty needle on the job? Does it change a nurse's life to help a patient deal with being the target of cruel stigmas? How does it feel to be a dentist who accepts patients who have been turned away from other dental offices? This is a medical illness that has taken on the persona of a social disease.

Much has been written by patients, families, and friends about the experience of living and dying with AIDS. Few stories, though, are told by professional caregivers who work with people with AIDS. Nurses, doctors, therapists, social workers, dentists, and others must help their patients cope with deteriorating bodies and all the pain, despair, and loss that this disease entails.

Acute bouts of illness can occur from day to day or even hour to hour. These quick changes interrupt scheduled appointments and require adjustments in the types of treatments that were planned. If a physical therapist plans a program based on the patient's needs, those needs abruptly change when the patient spikes a temperature of 104 degrees. Suddenly, the patient becomes very sick, and the treatment needs to be altered on the spot.

During the course of a work shift, health professionals may help patients come to terms with dying and death. The nature of death may be prolonged suffering, along with torment from societal stigmas, fears, and indignity. Naturally, it is painful to watch clients lose their mental and physical faculties and die. Some health care providers feel that they should have all of the answers, but instead come face-to-face with their own limitations. Many experience anxiety, exhaustion, burnout, or apathy.

How are these caregivers affected by working with people with AIDS?

The Search for Answers Begins

To find out what it's like for health professionals to care for people with AIDS, I went to the source. I spoke with men and women of varying ages and work experience. I sought caregivers who worked in a variety of clinical settings with patients from different walks of life, whose patients had gotten infected with HIV through intravenous drug use, sexual contact, both, or transmission from the mother during pregnancy. These caregivers included hetero-sexuals and homosexuals, Christians and Jews, people of color and whites, some experienced and some still learning the ropes.

We talked in public and private hospitals, offices, and a prison. I listened to an outpouring of satisfaction and heartache in air-conditioned offices with designer decor and behind bars with mice running around my feet and prisoners banging on the door. Caregivers shared their beliefs, attitudes, and feelings. They laughed. They cried. The tape recorder played on. Jessie, a prison social worker, added through tears, "Now that you've opened me up like this, what are you going to do to put me back together?!"

Although I came to each interview with a consistent list of questions, I tried to be flexible and go where I was being taken. I found it difficult to stand back and listen dispassionately. As I became more absorbed by the stories, I literally had to bite my tongue to keep my mouth shut! As they bared their souls, they thanked me for letting them give voice to their emotions — "I never realized this" and "I never told anybody this before."

These are the stories of ten health care professionals who work with people with AIDS.[1] I assigned fictitious names to maintain their anonymity. They tell us how they cope with loss and death on the job. To preserve the immediacy of each caregiver's experience, the stories are told from the point of view — and in the voice — of the individual caregivers who I interviewed. In their own words and through their personal and professional insights, we get to see what their work means to them. Through their eyes, ears, heads, and hearts, we get a rare, insider's view of life. This is a largely untold story whose time has come.

Do I get sucked in by what's happening to these people? Absolutely. But I no longer drive home in tears. I have recuperative powers that I didn't have two years ago.

Jessie, social worker

Chapter One

Understanding Acquired Immune Deficiency Syndrome (AIDS)

We're in more danger of getting other things like hepatitis or TB than we are of getting infected with HIV. TB's not diagnosed here until about a week after the patient is diagnosed with HIV. I'm not scared, but I think about it.

Jessie, social worker

AIDS is perhaps the most tragic epidemic of this century. It is now recognized that although AIDS was at first considered to be a "gay" disease, the human immuno-deficiency virus (HIV) affects people of all races, religions, ages, sexes, and sexual orientations. AIDS touches the lives of the people infected, along with their family and friends, co-workers, health care professionals, and the community at large. AIDS leaves its mark in every social strata. However, its horrible impact among disenfranchised populations, such as gay and bisexual men, people of color, and intravenous drug users, suggests that the disease and all of its ramifications is a "them, not us" problem.

A virus, one of the planet's simplest organisms, is the culprit that has transformed so many lives. This tiny entity has highlighted the social plights of urbanization and devastated the already poor economies of African and other Third World nations. The AIDS virus then flourished in industrialized countries, ultimately inspiring many to face the challenge of survival, while raising discrimination to new levels. New phrases entered the language, such as drug addiction and needle-sharing. With this awareness, extra-marital sexual relations, bisexuality, homosexuality, sexually transmitted, blood-borne, and bodily fluids are now parts of education campaigns aimed at high-risk behaviors. With AIDS rampant, one might anticipate that people would heed the warnings, but the disease continues to spread at a dizzying pace.

AIDS is a disease of loss and abandonment. It's not uncommon to lose a job, a home, or insurance. Friends and families often turn away and abandon the person with AIDS. It's a disease of fear and ignorance, sexism and racism, ostracism, loneliness, and rejection. Even many health care professionals shy away. It's a disease of physical and mental deterioration commonly occurring in a young population in the prime of life. It's a disease of guilt for having passed this "killer" to intimate partners or children. It's a disease of uncertainty because average life expectancies, average latency periods before symptoms appear, and frequency and types of opportunistic infections are unknown. It's a disease of expensive medications, care, and treatment.[1] Yet, it's also a disease of personal growth, of people reaching out to others and tirelessly helping and supporting those in need.

In the Beginning...

In 1981, the modern world of health care was about to face a challenge beyond its expectations. At the University of Los Angeles School of Medicine and at Cedars of Sinai Hospital in Los Angeles five young homosexual men were hospitalized with pneumocystis carinii pneumonia (PCP), an illness rarely seen in healthy young people. The men also developed other infections seen only in patients with severely depressed immune systems. These patients were reported in the *Morbidity and Mortality Weekly Report (MMWR)* of the Centers for Disease Control (CDC) in the United States.[2,3] A subsequent *MMWR* reported a high incidence of Kaposi's sarcoma (KS), another very unusual disease in a young and otherwise healthy population. From January 1979 to July 1981, there were twenty cases of KS in New York and six in California. All the patients were sexually active. Four had PCP *and* KS. Eight died within two years of the diagnosis.[4]

Even though 1981 is the year commonly acknowledged for the first cases of AIDS, there is evidence that HIV existed long before 1981. In Zaire, in central Africa, stored blood from as long ago as 1959 was found to have antibodies to HIV.[5] Among seventy-five serum samples from the west Nile district of Uganda, fifty were HIV-positive.[6]

In 1982, AIDS was discovered in groups other than homosexual men when intravenous drug users, Haitians, and hemophiliacs became ill. A twenty-month-old boy contracted AIDS in December 1982 from a blood transfusion. Later, one of the blood donors became ill with AIDS.[7] At the end of 1988, the World Health Organization (WHO) reported more than 124,000 cases of AIDS in 142 countries worldwide, estimating the actual number to be between 200,000 and 250,000.[8] Forty-nine countries reported more than fifty cases of AIDS.[9] Not all cases of this pandemic are accurately reported, especially in the developing nations, and the figures change continually.

By the end of December 1996, 573,800 people over thirteen years old in the United States had full-blown AIDS. At that time, single-mode exposure categories of transmission among adults and adolescents accounted for 79 percent (454,527) of the AIDS cases in this particular population of people with AIDS.[10] The Centers for Disease Control and Prevention issued these percentages of cases from a single mode of exposure:

> 48 percent men who have sex with men
> 21 percent injecting drug use
> 1 percent hemophilia/coagulation disorder
> 8 percent heterosexual contact
> 1 percent receipt of transfusion of blood or blood
>   component
> 0 percent (n=12) received a transplant of tissues,
>   organs, or artificial insemination
> 0 percent (n=80) other or undetermined.[11]

Multiple modes of exposure among adults and adolescents accounted for fourteen percent (78,735) of the AIDS cases among this segment of the AIDS population. Risk was not reported or identified in seven percent of the cases.[11]

The subtotal of AIDS cases in the United States for children under thirteen years old was 7,629 by December of 1996,[10] with exposure categories listed as:

90 percent mother with or at risk for HIV infection
5 percent receipt of blood transfusion, blood
    components, or tissue
3 percent hemophilia/coagulation disorder
2 percent undetermined.[12]

According to the CDC, from the time when the disease was first reported through December 1996, 357,598 adults and adolescents and 4,406 children under the age of thirteen have died from AIDS in the United States.[13]

Ninety percent of the Americans infected with AIDS are young men, and almost 75 percent are between the ages of twenty-five and forty-four.[14] For women between the ages of twenty-five and thirty-four, the major cause of death in New York City is AIDS-related problems, such as invasive cervical cancer and pulmonary tuberculosis. When the immune system is debilitated, it can't do its job to fight off marauding invaders like viruses, bacteria, fungi, yeast, and protozoa. The body becomes open to other diseases which may ultimately cause death.

In the United States, AIDS-related diseases are the leading cause of death for men between the ages of twenty-five and forty-four and the fourth leading cause of death for women in that age group. New York, California, Florida, Texas, and New Jersey, in descending order, are the states with the largest number of people with AIDS to date. Through December 1996, fifty-two health care workers have had documented HIV seroconversion, when antibodies to HIV appeared in their blood, following occupational exposure, twenty-four of whom subsequently developed AIDS.[15]

The number of AIDS cases is increasing among all racial and ethnic groups. Risk factors rather than ethnicity are the reasons people of color are affected more than three times as often as white people and why 75 percent of all the women with AIDS are black or Hispanic.[16] "Communities of color," such as African-American blacks, Haitian blacks, black West Indians, Latinos, Puerto Ricans, Cape Verdeans, Portuguese, and Asian Americans, have diverse cultures with different values and beliefs.[17] The taboo of homosexuality, homelessness, substance abuse, violence, illiteracy, and poverty can be barriers to AIDS education.

Compromises and Opportunities of the Immune System

Acquired immune deficiency syndrome is aptly named. The diseases are acquired and not inherited. The immune system is severely compromised, and it's a collection of diseases not just a single disease.[8]

AIDS is a syndrome which results from an infection caused by a retrovirus, the human immunodeficiency virus (HIV). Instead of deoxyribonucleic acid (DNA) as the genetic material which is in viruses, a retrovirus is a type of virus that has ribonucleic acid (RNA) as its genetic material and has an enzyme called reverse transcriptase, which makes a DNA-copy of its RNA. Viruses reproduce by themselves, but retroviruses utilize the host cells to reproduce. HIV primarily invades white blood cells, where it takes over the protein production of DNA and RNA. The white blood cell then produces the HIV's DNA instead of its own, reproducing the virus instead of reproducing itself.

Early diagnosis of HIV infection is virtually impossible, because the majority of the viral behavior takes place in the cells and not the blood. Consequently, the immune system doesn't become alerted to the infection, which may create a time lag of up to several months between the onset of the viral infection and the production of antibodies.[18] The virus may be dormant in the original cells up to six years or more before reproducing, creating another time lag between the initial infection and symptom identification.[19] Because this virus mutates, producing new strains that may be different from strains in antibody formation, it's difficult to fully comprehend incubation duration and medication effectiveness and ultimately achieve a stable approach to treatment and research.[20]

Transmission of HIV occurs through sexual contact, exposure to blood, blood products, or other bodily secretions through intravenous, subcutaneous, intramuscular, or mucosal routes, and perinatally from mother to infant.[21] Exposure to HIV-infected blood via a needlestick injury, contact with nonintact broken, cut, or chapped skin, or through mucous membranes, such as the eyes and mouth, are the modes of transmission of HIV to health care staff in the workplace.[15] A mucous membrane exposure or a skin opening is needed to permit the HIV to reach the bloodstream, and there must be enough virus in the transmitted fluid to actually infect the other individual. Transmission of the virus through sexual activity and intravenous drug activity with blood-contaminated needles are two of the most common methods for causing infections.[22] The HIV cannot be transmitted through casual contact or from sharing households, meals, or bathrooms.[23]

There is no direct test for AIDS at this time, but there are antibody tests that reveal the presence of HIV antibodies, which can be used as an indicator of the transition to illness. HIV affects the immune system, the central nervous system, certain blood cells, and every other organ system of the body. It can also cause heart disease, joint problems, and cancer.[24]

A person who has no symptoms of illness but who is HIV-infected is also known as being HIV-positive. As the immune system becomes further suppressed, the opportunity exists for various infections to develop. When these opportunistic infections appear, the individual develops full-blown AIDS. These infections can be protozoan, fungal, yeast, bacterial, or viral.

Symptoms of AIDS can include fever, fatigue, copious night sweats, and swollen lymph nodes. Because these symptoms may also indicate other bacterial or viral infections, the red flag for AIDS becomes their persistent nature (for example, lymphadenopathy or swollen lymph nodes in two or more areas, excluding the groin, for two or more weeks, weight loss of ten or more pounds over a few weeks that is not from dieting and exercise, or persistent fatigue not associated with physical or emotional stress).[1]

A cytomegalovirus infection, for example, may occur in the large bowel, resulting in abdominal pain and diarrhea. If this infection is in the lungs, the patient can have a cough and difficulty breathing. A person can feel burning and pain and have difficulty eating if the esophagus is affected. In the retina of the eyes, a cytomegalovirus infection can cause blurred and impaired vision and blindness.

Kaposi's sarcoma, one of the HIV-associated malignancies, is usually diagnosed by the appearance of purple-brown spots on the skin. Some people may have no other symptoms. Other patients may have a fast progression of the disease, affecting their lungs, heart, eyes, gastrointestinal tract, and other areas of their bodies.

Medical Illness or Social Disease

AIDS is not only physically devastating but also causes far-reaching psychological, emotional, and social ramifications for the people with AIDS and their families and friends. In a reversal of the natural order, parents are burying their children; babies, children, teenagers, young adults, and middle-aged adults with AIDS are facing their own premature death or that of their friends and loved ones. Unresolved issues, which might otherwise remain buried, rear their heads. Parents whose sons have chosen to lead clandestine, double lives, for example, may gain implied or actual knowledge of their son's sexual orientation when they learn of his diagnosis of AIDS.[25] Common themes of shock, anger, loss, and grief prevail among people with AIDS, along with concern for physical, emotional, and financial well-being.

The non-physical manifestations of the disease, which affect many people, do not leave the health care professionals unscathed. Professionals, assistants, and aides in medicine, dentistry, rehabilitation, nursing, and social work treat people with AIDS daily in a range of settings, such as hospitals, rehabilitation centers, private practices, outpatient clinics, and prisons. Much has been written about dealing with AIDS from the perspective of the people with AIDS, their families, and friends, but the professional care-givers are usually not heard from. When professionals discuss the fear, denial, anger, guilt, isolation, depression, withdrawal, rejection, and grief which people with AIDS may face, they usually fail to recognize that as caregivers, they, too, often face these same concerns.[26] Health care professionals who work with people with AIDS and spend their time amidst deterioration, dysfunction, dying, fear, prejudice, and stress have a story to tell and feelings and insights to share.

> *It's really a challenge to all aspects of my personality. I have to utilize all the skills I have as a physical therapist to do the best job that I can for them, knowing full well that the improvements that I make are only going to be on a short-term basis for most of these people.*
>
> Steve, physical therapist

Chapter Two

Jessie: From Terminal to Chronic Illness

I'm really good at helping people find the best part of the best. So, why not work with the worst! I can find hope in almost any situation.

At age 42, Jessie is a white, homosexual woman with twenty years experience as a social worker, including three working with people with AIDS. During her career, she has gravitated to work with people who nobody wants, those who have sunk to the bottom. In the past year, she has worked in a prison with more than 100 people with AIDS. Her tough exterior masks a heart of gold. She seems at ease meeting clients where they are and is not rattled by their reactions when she tells them that they're HIV-positive.

This job represents a progression in her relationship with many of her clients. She worked with several of the same people in a previous job where she sometimes had to remove children from their homes because of the parent's drug addiction. When she visits these people now in prison, it's old home week, but with even higher stakes.

When Jessie isn't working, she raises a twelve-year-old soccer-playing son, with her committed partner of almost twenty years, and is handy with a garden tiller and a hammer.

At the time of our discussion at her workplace, she was drinking her lunch — a powdered diet drink — and struggling with its regimen. Instantly we had something in common!

Perhaps because of her years of experience working with people with a host of social ills, she didn't seem distracted by the prisoners frequently banging on the door or the mice "dancing" in the room while we talked. I was.

Here is her account of working with AIDS patients behind bars.

Sexual Preference and Work

There are very few gay men here. When there is someone, I choose to work with him. I sort all the slips, and they're coded for risk factor — homosexual or bisexual. I've worked with the two couples we've had here. We had some guys who had long-term relationships inside the prison. I've worked with them a lot. One of the couples is positive, and one is negative. I'm not "out" on the job except to the woman with whom I work. It would just wreak havoc for a lot of people here.

A lot of the women are definitely lesbians and all are HIV-negative. I can pick and choose who gets a letter and who gets a face-to-face meeting when I give negative results. Some I'll choose to see because they have a lot of questions, like "is it true that we're the safest in this kind of sex?" I'd never tell them where I'm coming from, but I can say with such assurance how not to be at risk in a lesbian relationship. I think that's where it's the most fun. That's really the only place that my sexual preference comes into play.

There's a lot of "institutional" homosexuality. By that I mean they do it here, but the minute they're out, they'd never do it again. I find that intriguing with both the men and the women. I had to tell a guy last week that he was infected. He was halfway through a sex change. He had very nice breasts, still had his penis, and was very cute. He was also Spanish so I couldn't talk directly with him. The interpreter said that he had been in a long-term relationship and felt that he had no risk. Having found out that he was HIV-positive was blowing him to pieces. Once in a while, you get interesting twists like that.

The prison is not a place to be "out." They're very red-necked. The guys who come in here who are effeminate get raped, attacked, beaten up. It's not the place to be open about your homosexuality.

My sexual preference was ultimately responsible for picking this specialty. My gay friends who died or who are ill with this disease got me into the work in the first place. They're the reason that I'm even doing this. If you were to take a poll, you'd find a lot of gay men and lesbians doing AIDS-related social work.

As a social worker, I could be doing a lot tamer things and be in a position where there is no risk. I think the key that drives people to work with HIV-positive or AIDS people is some twist in their personality or a personal hook.

A lot of women nurses and social workers I know working in this field are lesbians. There must be a piece of us that thinks that even if we're not open about our sexuality, we're contributing to the lives of people with a sexual preference that gets put down a lot.

We're all doing this for some reason. We chose it. We're good at it, and we're compassionate. I do it because I do it well, and I'm willing to do it. But it does take its toll.

Maintaining Emotional and Physical Health

We vent a lot here. It's built into the support that we have. When I leave here, I never think about it again. Some nights, I'm extremely annoyed to see the news or a flash that comes on TV that says, "Data report: The World Health Organization says there will be twenty million infected people by the year 2000." I'm annoyed because it brings me back to thinking about it.

I usually head from work to the soccer field to watch my son play. I'm busy every night, and I intentionally don't take reading material home with me. If I have research or something HIV-related to do, I do it here. I try to separate what I think about during the day from at-night stuff and weekend stuff.

If I choose not to see three people today because I'm not feeling up to it emotionally, I can do that. Part of taking care of myself is working within the system such that I don't overkill when I don't have to. Don't get me wrong. There are plenty of things to do, but it's not the kind of environment that puts pressure on you to rush with the paperwork.

If I'm having a bad day, I take care of myself on the job. I might take the whole afternoon and go to the library to read about drug addiction because I'm working with a particular woman. I have freedom to do that. On other jobs, you don't get to take care of yourself as well.

I'm doing a lot of gardening at home, which is a scary thought because I hate gardening, but all of a sudden, I'm in up to my neck. Gardening puts me back in touch with the physical component of working off some of the pressures. Walking and jogging weren't enough to push me to the level of physical exhaustion. I found new forms of using my body. The day I worked with a problem inmate, I went home and made lawn where there was no lawn before. I almost passed out from heat exhaustion, but I'm sure I worked out some of the stress physically.

I also feel very good about the work I'm doing here. I get positive feedback, which always helps with the whole emotional impact of working with people with AIDS.

Coming Up Through the Ranks

After years of working with mothers in child welfare, I find myself working with the same clientele here. Three years ago, I took kids away from three of the women who are here now. These women were habitual drug users and are now HIV-positive. A couple of the men here are the fathers of some of those kids. I'm seeing the same people, which makes it easier to relate to some of their needs. On top of layers of poverty, drug use, and the multi-problem family situation, you add a layer of a terminal disease. They didn't have enough wherewithal to solve their other problems before. Now, they're overwhelmed. In their eyes, now that they have a terminal disease, there's no way they'll get their kids back. There's no reason to try to get their act together.

I think the reason that I've survived is that I came up through the ranks, working at one particular problem or another. The work doesn't depress me, although it's harder to find hope with these people than it was before. Before, I could use their kids or some other things to motivate some of the women. Now, they realize they're not going to live long enough to see their kids grow up, so there's no point.

Finding that Little Speck — Challenges of the Job

Working with this population, I'm challenged to find the one thing — the critical element for each person — that will get them past how they feel about having a chronic disease to make plans for their future. When I tell someone that he or she is HIV-positive, the first reaction is that their life is over. The biggest challenge is not getting the words out of my mouth, it's getting these people to refocus. I want them to understand that they have a chronic disease, perhaps not a terminal one, and that the quality of their lives can go on even though they're HIV-positive.

If it were me, I would have other things in my life to look forward to. These people are already at the bottom. They're in jail for prostitution, drug abuse, or selling drugs. They already don't see a lot of reason to live. The challenge is to help them look at their lives in a different way. If they're totally depressed, what's to stop them from returning to drugs the minute they're released? Every day of their incarceration, the women say, "I can't wait to get out of here so I can get high." Getting high for these people will kill them. My challenge is to find that little speck in a person that allows them to refocus.

Twists to their Life Stories — Feeling Overwhelmed

Last month, for three weeks in a row, I only had to tell a few people that they were HIV-positive. We were doing a lot of education. That's a very upbeat part of the job because people want to know how to stay negative. Certainly, as a public health specialist, the whole focus of this job is to support the people who are positive and reach the people who are negative but still at high risk. Sometimes, I get absolutely overwhelmed. Last week alone, I told three women and two men they were positive. The women were either young or pregnant or had a lot of kids at home. Every day of the week, I was telling somebody that he or she was infected. What a strain!

It was incredibly draining because they all had different twists to their life stories. One woman was a twenty-two-year-old call girl, who was very articulate. She really understood when I told her about her medical problems. She was in the wrong place at the wrong time. She had protection and was doing all the right things. She was very upwardly mobile and came from a strong family. This woman could have been me.

I feel that I'm not making much progress a lot of the time, but I'll take the little improvements. That twenty-two-year-old woman had a boyfriend. He came in for a family session. It was encouraging to me that he could face the fact that she was HIV-positive and that he seemed to accept that he would have to wear a condom for the rest of his life if he married her.

As time goes by, the actual pain decreases. There was a thirty-one-year-old black woman, with three children who have been in the custody of the Department of Children, Youth, and Families [DCYF] for two years. She was about to lose permanent custody of them, and she knew that. She came to prison on a Monday. On Tuesday, a doctor told her she had syphilis. On Wednesday, they told her that she was pregnant, and on Thursday morning, I told her she was HIV-positive. She was overwhelmed by the amount of news.

A couple of people overheard me giving her options and accused me of pushing abortion as the best alternative. I was fighting with my own emotions about abortion and I wondered if I really had pushed it. Was I thinking, deep down inside, that because she had a fifty–fifty chance of producing an HIV-positive baby, the best solution was abortion?

The woman was your typical, multi-problem mother who really never made any decisions in her life. Somebody else always made them for her. To describe why she was in here this time, she told me, "I signed the contract with DCYF, and I promised them no more drugs and no more prostitution."

"How did you get in here?"

"Well, it wasn't my fault. The guy who propositioned me was a cop."

"You got here because you agreed to have sex with him."

"But it was a cop."

"But just by the fact that you agreed to have sex with him, you broke your contract even though you knew it would impact on getting your kids back."

She couldn't see the connection. The nurses and doctors definitely felt that termination of pregnancy was right for this woman because she had other medical issues.

She had three children to reunite with and that, strictly speaking, would be the best answer for her. My job was to relay this information to her and work with her one-to-one.

Through her indecision, she made her decision because, before long, it was too late for termination of pregnancy. There was no way to pay for it, anyway. I would have had to raise the money because the prison system doesn't pay for abortions. It would have had to come from some place like the state AIDS project. That kind of case takes a lot out of me.

This was particularly bad because it was tough to tell her. She was already devastated from the other news. She was already not able to hold it together on her own, and now she had to live with a chronic illness and try to get her kids back. Her first thought was that if DCYF found out about her HIV they wouldn't give the kids back to somebody who is HIV-positive. That's not true. That would be blatant discrimination. I know, because my last three cases were discrimination cases against people who were HIV-positive.

Some of the meetings take less time because the people don't want to see you again, they don't want to be seen with you, or they don't want to discuss it. With some of them, you get one hour to give them all the medical and prevention information and to get out of them any names of people who might need to be tested. Half the people we see are getting out the next day. So it's a one-shot thing.

There have been mistakes made in this unit. In one case, somebody wasn't told that he was positive, he went home on furlough and slept with somebody and put them at risk. When other people are put at risk, it certainly can overwhelm you.

Experience is a Good Teacher

They wouldn't hire anybody to do this job who wasn't at least forty. I had already worked with the worst clientele. Taking kids from mothers is probably the next toughest thing to telling somebody they have a terminal disease. Even though I came into this with some age and experience, it's still hard. When I walk away after telling someone about the infection, it's really difficult, but the devastation is not as great as it used to be. After telling ten people they were HIV-positive, I was having a real hard time. After telling seventy-five people, the adrenaline rush was still there for me trying to get the words out. Nobody has reacted violently, but the men's reactions ran the gamut from "so what" to saying "I'm going to cry. Is that ok?" I've actually sat with someone for an hour, and he said nothing. I've learned that no matter how they react, I can adjust to that reaction, and it will be okay. Two years ago, I didn't know that.

Today, I know more about the disease than I did before, and I am able to answer their questions in a more reassuring way. I know people who are alive after fifteen years, and I have seen people who are ten years into the virus without any major symptoms. I have seen the people. I know them.

Still, we have somebody die every two months. We have people in the hospital now who are really close to death. When I look back on my first terminal client at another agency four years ago, I remember someone asking me, "Are you ready for her to die?" At the time, I answered, "Die?" Today, I'd answer yes. Actually, death would be a relief for a lot of these people.

Feeling Effective, Feeling Gratified

I remember a woman who was married to a fisherman. She was already out of prison when we got the test results. I sent her a letter telling her I needed to talk to her. She called immediately. I chose to tell her in her own home. She was very responsible. She gave me names of everybody who needed to be tested.

I spent about two hours with her, and before I knew it, there were five other women from the apartment building in this woman's living room. They all shared the same needle when they did drugs, so they were all very concerned. Her husband called from his fishing ship which was about 200 miles off the coast. He was nearly hysterical, but I was able to communicate with all these people, get all the other women to the right resources, get all of them tested, reassure them about the facts, talk to the husband over the phone, reassure him about the kids, and set up an appointment for a test for him.

Ultimately, this family stayed with me even though they were out of prison. We did some family therapy. In the end, nobody else in the apartment building tested positive, but both the husband and wife were HIV-positive. They were asymptomatic and very willing to try to give up the drugs and to connect with the doctors. I had some effect on their family life and their sticking together. They had small kids and had to learn the risks. If they kept doing IV drugs, they wouldn't see their kids get any older. They both enrolled in an outpatient drug program and followed through with that.

Even though this was a difficult case, I really felt effective because I had the resources they needed. They used them. They came back here. There were no hidden agendas. A lot of the guys leave here, go home to their families, and never tell anybody that they are HIV-positive. Working with this couple was one of the more gratifying cases and probably the most effective that I'm ever going to be. And that only happened once. One little apartment building on one little street got the facts and knew about their risks. Sadly, about a year later, we had six fishermen off the same boat who all turned out to be HIV-positive.

Lip Service and Other Deeds — Feeling Ineffective

I'm thinking of four women, two of whom are dead, two of whom are on the street now. When they were in prison, they used all the medical facilities, took their AZT, went to the education classes on drug abuse, talked a really good story. We spent a lot of time getting them housing so that they wouldn't return to the scene of the crime with relatives or friends who do drugs all the time. We set them up with a doctor on the outside. We got them supplemental income and medical assistance.

I've had three cases like one with a woman who was released on a Sunday. I don't work on Sundays so I wasn't able to drive her to the apartment that I had arranged for her. I asked the nun who worked with this woman and who comes on Sunday to drive the woman to the apartment. When the nun went to pick her up, the woman was already gone. She never showed up at the apartment, although she knew where it was. She never went to the doctor. Even if I had been here to drive her to the apartment, she probably would have been gone two hours later. Chances are, like the other two women, she's back into doing IV drugs. She weighed sixty pounds the last time she was admitted to the hospital. This time, if she's not picked up right away, it will kill her. That's what happened to the other two women.

A lot of this job is doing discharge planning with women who, from the minute they are handed their plastic bag and step outside the door, are not going to follow through on what we set up. It was a hard lesson for me two years ago when that first woman died. Everybody was working on her behalf, from the judge on down. She went straight back to doing drugs and died on the streets. Nothing makes you feel less effective than hearing that someone died or was admitted to the hospital from an overdose after they had been in drug treatment all the time they were in jail. That's typical of the cases we have.

"Why Am I Doing This?" — Anger and Frustration

When I'm overwhelmed by the paperwork on my desk, feeling ineffective and not wanting to do any more, I start to question why I'm in this line of work. Some of the nurses, or other people who are already burned out, tell me what a fool I am for even caring. In turn, I'll get passive-aggressive and do something to mess up their schedules, such as not showing up at a meeting or something like that. Then anger grows on top of that. Frustration, too.

It seems that no matter what I do, it's not going to work out in the client's best interest. I ultimately end up questioning myself as to why I chose to do this work.

This week, we've been working on a number of

grants to get money to do discharge planning. Once again, I see the hope. I don't get in the pits for very long.

Carelessness and Needlesticks

If a staff member sticks himself and is at risk, we're called in to talk to him. We have a lot of nurses who don't wear gloves and who are always in a hurry. One nurse stuck herself three times with an HIV-positive needle in my presence. Three times!

The first time, it was devastating. But because I was there and I knew the resources, I knew that if she wanted AZT as a preventative, she had to take it right at that moment. Because I was right there to advise her, an incredible bond formed with that staff member. One guy has been stuck three times, and I've been there two out of the three times. I never walk into that dispensary without hugging him. He's not even a guy that I have much in common with — except we've shared every test result.

There are so many needlestick incidents for one main reason — caregivers are careless, very careless! Some of the clients, though, have such track marks that if they pull away at all, it's very easy for the nurse to get stuck because the needle is so low. But all of the needlesticks that I've witnessed have been total, absolute carelessness. They either dropped the needle or carried it in the wrong way to the vacutainer so that when it dropped, it stuck in their hand.

One time, I was in the middle of doing paperwork as two nurses were going as fast as they could to give TB tests to lines of inmates. They were using one vacutainer to get rid of the needles. They met right in front of me. One nurse stuck the other, and the guy she had just done was a known HIV-positive. We all looked at each other. The nurse who had been stuck went on AZT, which made him very sick.

I've learned a lot of medical things that I never had to know before. We no longer do anything unless everybody has their own needle vacutainer. Get rid of your own needles. Don't touch anyone else's. I have now gone every-where where babies come to visit. I put out hazardous waste containers for the diapers and gloves for people who don't know the infant. I have placed universal precaution signs everywhere to get people to use the containers if they're not already.

If we get an HIV-positive test result, we're required to notify the person within twenty-four hours. If we can't, we have to turn the matter over to another agency. There's something about getting somebody's positive result on your desk ... and they always seem to come in on Friday. I'll never take a Friday off. We can't let ourselves go home until the person has been notified, even though it's not a matter of state law. We simply won't leave before telling them, even if it means that we stay until six o'clock.

I've had to learn on the job how to decrease the risk for people. That's been a more satisfying part of my job because nobody here wants to learn all the itsy-bitsy rami-fications and the statistics of knowing that only four out of fifteen hundred health care workers who stick themselves have ever turned positive. They only want that statistic after they've stuck themselves. If that happens, they know who they can call. I'm a resource. That's the good part of the job — until somebody becomes positive.

Fears, Common Sense, and Transmission

When I've done stupid things like going to a hospital and talking within two feet of somebody who is diagnosed with active TB a day later, I realize that I don't think all the time. I'm also a toucher. I touch people whose rash is everywhere, and I'm not a real good hand-washer. I've had to change my way of taking care of myself. Now, I wash my hands immediately. I haven't stopped touching, but I realize that although I'm not afraid of getting it, I have a healthy respect for this virus.

In some cases, I've probably put myself at risk. I used to carry a lot of blood samples to the lab in paper lunch bags. One slip on my part, and I would either land on the glass or splatter blood. In order to be more careful, I now bring plastic lunch containers. If my clients are really anxious, I offer them another test. To get the results immediately, I'll take the sample to the lab myself. So now I use a little lunch bucket. If I drop it, there's less risk. I think about that a lot.

In my support group, we talk a lot about putting ourselves at risk, and I've never taken it to heart like some of the people in my unit. Some of the people can get swollen glands and a sore throat, and immediately they think they're HIV-positive. So we joke about that. We also have a test every six months. I don't consider myself personally or professionally at risk, yet there's a piece of me that says I work with this every day and come into contact with the blood, and even though I'm careful ... so I keep getting the test. There's a part of me that must want reassurance.

Last week, right after I told a woman that she was positive, she got hit in the face with a piece of furniture. Blood was spewing everywhere. I don't know if the nurses knew about the woman's HIV, but they were pretty good and grabbed gloves anyway. There were other people in the dispensary, and blood was hitting everywhere. The possibility of getting it on your eyelid or in your eye was there, and everyone was at risk. These places are notorious for not having their bleach on hand. I personally ordered gallons of bleach and put them in every dispensary because when I need it, I need to know it's there.

The Uncertainty, the Unknown

Every case is different with this disease. I've told people that they were positive, and they died three months later. I always hope that the people who I've told will lead long lives, but there are some who were really sick before they came here. Another factor of uncertainty is the test itself. I once told somebody that he was positive, and a second test came back negative six months later. In the past two weeks, I've had two tests come back as "indeterminate." According to the textbook, these cases should be seroconverting from negative to positive, yet the tests came back negative. A year ago, if a result was indeterminate, and two tests out of four tests were positive, I could say that the antibodies were probably waiting to react to the virus. I can't say that any more.

I told one woman that she was positive, and she was on the streets thinking that she was positive. Another test came through six months later and said she was negative. I couldn't find the woman. It took me three months to track her down. If I had to pick a high point of this job, it was telling that woman, on the steps of her tenement house, that she was indeed negative. Upon hearing the good news, this woman just grabbed me and cried for a half hour. It was like Christmas!

We don't know what the course of this disease will be, when there will be a vaccine, or which drugs work the best. So much is still unknown. AIDS is not like cancer, which runs a more familiar course.

I Was So Naive — What I've Learned

I've learned that nobody has split over an HIV-positive diagnosis. In cases where I thought the negative spouse would be totally flabbergasted and want to leave, I've seen the family unit come together in a stronger way. Mothers will call me who haven't spoken to their incarcerated children for years, asking how serious this is and how they could be the most supportive. I didn't expect to learn that.

I've learned that the people I think are going to be the weakest and take it the hardest, often end up being the strongest. I've learned that street walkers and sex workers are very strong, survival-oriented women. In helping them plan about their future career, they seem very capable of finding all the resources and believe that condoms work. If they do stay in the business, they will double up on condoms. I've found them to be more resourceful and stronger than I previously thought.

I think the biggest problem I'm having now is working with people who are getting closer to death and haven't come to terms with life and dying. I'm searching for that ultimate answer to help people be at peace with themselves. I've learned that many people prefer to take major drugs and be out of it in their last few months of life rather than suffer pain. I'm not sure I would choose that option.

I've learned that denial is an incredible phenomenon. I've got guys who deny their infection to themselves and others. It doesn't become a reality for them. That's really scary because I know they'll go out and sleep around. They point blank tell me, "Listen, somebody gave this to me. What's the difference if I pass it on?" I think that's totally irresponsible. All I can do is give them the facts.

Whether it's the john on the street or the woman who becomes this guy's girlfriend, we have to approach this disease from a specific point — if you get sexually involved with somebody, you are ultimately putting yourself at risk, and you have to take precautions and responsibility. I used to think that all people would be responsible. What a fool! I was so naive!

People are egocentric. I've watched men share needles in prison a day after I told them they were HIV-positive. I can't do anything else. When I have two or three cases like that in a row, I head back to the women. I find that women are much more considerate of other people, but devastating to themselves. There are women on the streets who won't share needles any more but still pump themselves full of drugs. In my experience, women have been more responsible about reporting sexual contacts, protecting their families, and telling their boyfriends. Any family contact that I've had has come through a woman.

I've also learned that I'm culturally ignorant. I've reported test results to Hispanics or Cambodians without realizing that in other cultures men never discuss sex with women. I have a twenty-year-old Cambodian man who is now on the street. I set up an appointment with an interpreter. When I explained to the interpreter what I wanted him to do, the interpreter said, "No way, he'll kill me." This man still walks the street while we talk. I'm sure he got HIV from a sex worker, and I'm sure that he's still spreading it around because nobody in his culture will tell him the news.

I've learned other things about myself. I know I'm compassionate. It's not a term that I always used about myself because my exterior can be pretty rigid, friendly but protected. I already knew that I was outgoing, competent, and serious about what I do. Working with HIV people has helped me realize that I'm also compassionate and sincere and able to let people be where they are.

I hear that some people are able to do this job for only two or three years. I can see myself in a different job, but not yet. I'm still learning every day. The whole piece of death and dying and helping at that end stage is just opening up. We have people here who were told by staff five or six years ago that they were infected. Now, they're dying.

"Why Do You Do This?"

People ask me why I do this. Every job I've ever had and liked has had a risk factor involved — confronting a mother about taking her kids out of her arms and taking them away or walking into the projects in a neighborhood where people didn't want white women. There's the same kind of adrenaline rush that comes from getting ready to tell somebody about their positive blood test. There's a personal hook for me that neither allows me to tire of the job nor stop seeing it as a challenge. Every time I have one of those test results slips in my hand, it pushes me to the limit of doing it to the best of my ability. That's a part of why I do it.

I need the challenge of what this does for me and the unknown of how somebody is going to react when I tell them. Sometimes, it's very easy. Somebody will say, "I knew this. I was diagnosed three months ago."

"How come you didn't tell the nurses here?"

"'Cause I don't think it's any of their business."

Or the patient's story where all the pieces start to unfold. You never know.

I like the unknown piece. It's exciting being on the cutting edge. Do I tell my people now that we're closer to getting a vaccine than we were two years ago? Absolutely. I use the term "chronic illness" now. Two years ago, I used "terminal illness." That's a big step forward.

I see this population as very needy. It must help me to work with needy people. There are so many things I can do that can be helpful. I'm also very comfortable with people who are, in their own terms, "victims." I have this crazy piece of me that can find hope in every situation. People keep asking me how long they have to live. I always answer, "as long as you want" because I know they can have a major impact on their own lives.

Innocence vs. Guilt

The media's distinction between innocence and guilt really annoys me. I don't care what somebody's behavior was. Nobody deserves this virus. A lot of people, including people who work here, ask why we're wasting all of this medical money on these people. They don't deserve it. They don't take care of themselves on the outside. They did drugs. They got what they asked for. My bottom line is that nobody deserves this. I don't care how they got it.

There have only been two people that I've had a hard time treating. One guy infected two of his children by molesting them, and another guy got three women pregnant after he knew he was positive. I didn't stop working with them, but I was aware of how I felt at the time I was talking to them. In my mind, they crossed the boundaries, but they still had the right to know the information. I just wasn't going one ounce further than necessary.

Staff Support Makes a Difference

I'm in a very supportive situation here. We have psychologists who work with us. You can either go in or they'll find you. The reason that we come back to the office at three or four is to talk over anything that was tough for us during the day. We have support groups with others who are doing the same thing that we're doing and who hash through the same kind of stuff. It's usually among the three of us within our unit. And that's enough for now. In the beginning, the administrators were more worried about us and had a psychologist assigned to our unit. It's a very different kind of world for state service.

We don't go home before talking about it! Compared to my past jobs, I rarely need to talk about work at home because I vent here. It's very unusual, but our boss believes it's the kind of support that we need.

I think I'm not burned out here because I get a lot of support. I like the professional freedom that I have. Sometimes when I feel very ineffective, my boss sends me home for a couple of days. You can't ask for better than that.

Chapter Three

Marlene: Endless Needs and Exhaustion

*I feel very enlightened by my patients and emotion-
ally moved. I tell them this, but I don't think they believe
me. I'm encouraged by the way people, who know that
they're dying and have terrible stress around them, have
such a vigor for life. It's very uplifting for me. Not all the
time, though.*

As a physician, Marlene has been working with
people with AIDS during her entire eleven year career.
Thirty-six years old, she is a white, heterosexual woman
who divides her time between cancer patients in a private
center and AIDS patients in a long-term state hospital.
During the past twelve months, she has worked with more
than 100 AIDS patients.

Her patients with AIDS are from low socioeconomic
and educational levels of life. Many are prisoners getting
treatment in this public facility. A significant number have a

history of intravenous drug use. Marlene had thought that she had very little in common with this patient population and has been surprised to see how much in common she does have.

Marlene is also the wife of a physician. Her husband has a hard time with the idea of gay men and says that may be why he doesn't do AIDS work. When Marlene talks about gay patients or colleagues, he gets more uptight. She's also the mother of two active preschool children and tries to be involved in the community. Like so many working women, it's always a challenge to balance work, children, husband, and household. It's hard to find time to rejuvenate herself. She enjoys antiquing and the ballet, both of which she has rarely done since she's had children.

Marlene is also a second-generation Holocaust survivor. Ever since she was a little girl, she's had a very strong sense of social responsibility, justice, and giving back to people. She remembers hearing about the people who risked their lives to help her parents and has never forgotten. This is her story.

Giving Back

I sometimes feel like it's a plague. I'd feel guilty if I turned my back on my patients and their families, but not only because I'd be turning away from my expertise. I think of a few of my friends and my parents who survived the Holocaust, and I feel that this is my test to do something. To make a mark, to say that I didn't just stand by and watch something happen and not take an active role in helping people.

What made some people help my parents and others not? How could people not have helped and just stood by? How could I just stand back in a different crisis — AIDS — and not be a part of the process of helping? In life, you're either a watcher or a doer. I'd feel guilty to say that I'm not a doer in this AIDS epidemic. My parents, however, are not thrilled. They view it as a tremendous risk to me, but I actually don't.

AIDS and Me — The Early Years

People who don't work with AIDS patients think there's a major difference between people with AIDS and people without AIDS. When I first started working with patients who had AIDS, I realized the difference very gradually. Those of us who worked in the early part of the epidemic in New York and San Francisco didn't know we would become medically historic.

When patients came into the hospital, we really didn't know what was happening with all of these young people. As house officers, residents, and physicians, we were very intrigued by this disease. Now, anyone would clearly recognize the problem as AIDS, but we didn't know back then. In the beginning, it was a natural part of my work day and, actually, a very interesting part of it. In internal medicine, we tended not to see young people sick in the hospital. I naturally gravitated to taking care of these young people who had a disease that we really didn't know much about. AIDS care was very frustrating. We didn't have a lot of treatment, and we didn't have a lot of the options that we have now.

I look back at the early period and realize that I never saw my work as an issue of choice. I never asked myself how I felt. I just did my work, and it was a very exciting thing to do. When I moved from New York to Washington, the epidemic hadn't really hit Washington, D.C. yet. All of a sudden, I realized that I had expertise in something that I hadn't realized was even an area in which to be an expert. Identifying the problems and taking care of patients who had a disease which was later recognized as AIDS, I had this experience which many of my colleagues did not share. It was the natural thing for me to continue taking care of patients who had AIDS. To do otherwise would be to throw away my experience.

Making Choices

I think people have to make a more active choice today to take care of AIDS patients. Back then, I just did it. At that time, I was already dealing with many of the issues of oncology — dying, internal disease process, and family issues — so it was a natural progression to work with AIDS. I ended up going into oncology, and the issues of quality of life that attracted me in the early years are still very important to me.

In the last few years, AIDS care has become less natural for me because the issues, problems, and frustrations are so apparent that they hit you on the head. You have to actively ask yourself why you're doing this. With eleven years of experience, it's even harder to turn my back on this clinical experience and all of the time that I have devoted.

I teach at the medical school, and the students come work with me. I have infectious disease fellows training under me, and I see that, to them, it's much more of an active choice. With me, it was different. I happened to be in

New York, and I happened to be attracted to the emotional side of patient care. The reason I went into oncology is probably the same reason I ended up continuing in AIDS work. It's the draw of providing emotional support for people who are sick. One might say that I could have gone into psychiatry, because the fact is I enjoyed the emotional support aspects of patient care.

Learning and Appreciating

In helping people go through these crises, I have grown in many ways. Most people look at this work as a burden. I think it's kind of a mixed bag, privilege and burden.

As a mother, I see the reality. The whole spectrum of life can become so abbreviated. We see this in medicine. Because I do oncology, I see people dying. Unfortunately, I see young people dying, too. The majority of my patients are my own age. I've learned how important it is just to enjoy your life. Life is short, and for some people, it's a lot shorter than they ever expected. So I think that I play a little bit harder when I'm not at work, and I enjoy my family a little bit more. I feel a little more sadness as well. I don't take life for granted as much as I might have if I hadn't seen what I've seen.

When I see young children who don't have any parents, I appreciate my kids a lot more. I never thought I'd ever say to my children that "there are children who have no food" and that sort of thing that I now say. When I was a kid, I didn't know "them." All those starving children in India didn't mean anything to me. Now I say to my family, "These are real people, you know. You don't realize how lucky you are." They'll probably say "Mommy doesn't know what she's talking about."

I appreciate much more the gift of being a health care worker. We've made tremendous strides in the medications and treatment of this disease and its infections. In addition to the gifts we give of the medicines, we have the ability to make people feel good about themselves and to embrace them and their partners. I appreciate the skills of my colleagues and that increases as time goes by.

I am more aware than I wanted to be of dying, and I think about it a lot. AIDS has a significant impact on a family, and it's not just the stigma. With my cancer patients, their partners don't get sick because my patient has cancer. They may be emotionally distraught, but they don't have the risk of getting sick. Outside of some familial cancers, their children are not going to get sick. With my AIDS patients, this may not be the case. We're talking about the family and the risk to the family. I end up appreciating my life more.

I appreciate the sexual freedom that I had twenty years ago that young kids who I counsel don't have. I appreciate the ability that I have in terms of my marriage that I won't have to deal with issues that many of my patients have to face. I appreciate that I can have children. I counsel a lot of women not to have children, although many of them still have children. So I appreciate more the freedom I have.

I realize the nameless undercurrent that exists in society. Hundreds of people easily fall into the statistics of AIDS, and I'm really struck by that. If I hadn't done AIDS work, I could have been blissfully unaware of the problems that are seen in the minority population. It's very ironic. In medical school, I actively chose not to end up in a public health care system, and here I am. This is the final irony because I felt very frustrated that society really was not going to be able to heal all the other problems that brought people to us, even though we could help people medically. Now I do what I chose not to do fifteen years ago, and the same frustration is there. I see that society still doesn't completely embrace all the other problems.

AIDS is kind of a chichi issue now. It's nice to do marches for AIDS and to raise money for AIDS, but the patients are not such a chichi population anymore — the minority population, the people with heavy drug use. I doubt whether foundations and celebrities will embrace this population as much and really work hard to heal some of the other issues. Friends who go to Africa and work with African patients often feel the same. It's the world that is being decimated, and it doesn't really make the news the same way. When Rock Hudson died of AIDS, people were devastated. The equally devastating stories that I encounter don't make the front page. This is the reality. There is a time in your life when you are somewhat idealistic and think that people feel bad and do a bit more. But the nature of the human beast is perhaps not as sympathetic as I would like to think.

I've learned how important health care teams are. Medicine is often very doctor-oriented, but I'm happy to say that I have always embraced nurses, social workers, drug counselors, and all the other parts of the team. All too often, they don't get credit for what they do. As a director of the unit, I try very hard to acknowledge everyone and that every component of health care is important. So much attention is paid to drugs that have been developed, but the people who wash the patients, do the sheets, and sit and feed people need to get equal credit.

I'm much more aware of the system of health care, and I wouldn't have been as aware if I didn't do AIDS work. Even in my cancer work, it seems very doctor-oriented. People come in, I give them chemo, and I spend time with them. The rest of their life is much more in order, and the pyramid of health care doesn't seem as apparent to me.

I've learned that it can suck you up to the point that, even though you're exhausted, you still feel that you can do more, but you can't. Patients need so much, and you have to realize that you can't do everything. Not only do you not have the cure, but you want them not to make "cure" the goal. I talk about quality of life, and I try hard to meet the patient's goals. People get very depressed when they put cure as the goal and don't reach the goal. No one is cured. Most of my cancer patients are not cured. My AIDS patients are not cured. So I set my battle a little bit differently, but it's easy to get sucked up.

The patients suck you up with all the problems of their lives. I don't know whether I let them suck me up or whether they just suck me up anyway.

"It's just this paper...."

"Could you get housing for me?"

"Could you do this...?"

"My family needs help."

It's just endless, and you know you could spend twenty-four hours a day on non-medical needs alone. When people die, do you go to their funerals? Do you spend time with their families? It's a never-ending need.

Intravenous drug users, in particular, have endless needs. They have a way of sucking you up into every problem of their lives such that you're totally spent. I've learned it's easy to get spent very quickly, and I've learned that I'm terrible at saying "no" to patients. I'm a good hit for every problem. I've learned that I probably couldn't run for politics. I just couldn't say "no" to any constituent. I've learned that I need to set better boundaries, and it's hard to do that. It's hard in AIDS because I feel guilty that people really are sick, but I have learned that I better set boundaries or I won't have anything left for myself.

Drawing the Line

I think that pediatric AIDS workers are a unique group of people. I did a short rotation in pediatric oncology, but it was overwhelmingly sad for me. The sadness is when people don't have a chance to live. If a child doesn't ever have a chance to live, it's even sadder. When I did pediatric oncology, I was pregnant, and I would come home devastated every night. As devastated or frustrated as I might feel at times with AIDS patients, I've never felt as sad as I did when I was taking care of a four-year-old with cancer who was dying. I am not actively volunteering to join the pediatric AIDS forces.

A Small Part of a Big Tragedy

Most people, who don't do what we do, constantly dwell on talking about how "it must be so sad." It is sad at times, and there are many times that I am very sad about what has happened to someone.

For some, I think death is a tremendous part of the process, and I don't view it as a terrible tragedy when they finally die. The tragedy happened many times before that if they didn't have a chance to live — particularly public health patients. It's such a tragedy when young women get

infected from their boyfriends or whatever. The women
never had a chance to live. Or the intravenous drug users
whose lives have been tragedies. AIDS is just a small part
of a big tragedy. When one person who has had this incredibly sad life can manage to get to the clinic on time and say
"happy birthday" to me or ask me how my day is, I find that
life-affirming. I know it sounds like a little nothing, but if
they can do that, wow!

The Ties that Bind

There is a certain positive side when people, despite
all the tragedy, still can enjoy their children, their family,
the basic relationships between their parents, although
many relationships are strained. There's so much in their
lives that is similar to my life. I actually laugh that there's
much more similarity than most people who don't do this
work would like to think.

People say to me, "You have nothing in common
with all those people you take care of." The irony is that a
lot of minority groups push for minority health care workers
to take care of this population. I'd love to see more minority
people doing this, but it's not happening.

I find that I have a lot in common with everyone,
and most people wouldn't say that. They'd say, "Oh, she's
not black, she's not Spanish, she's not this." They're my
patients. I love them, and they love me. Our differences
really don't make any difference.

There is a positive side to AIDS care that people
from the outside don't really think about or understand. It's
the zest for living that many of these people have. There's
one guy who says that everyone is just living and breathing

AIDS, but he says, "I am living and breathing life." I get so uplifted by him. He's had AIDS for almost four years now. He's a very active person who enjoys every minute. I don't envy that he will probably die before I do, but I do envy his enthusiasm.

My Challenges

Academically, I find AIDS care challenging. I teach, and it's a challenge to be exciting to medical students and to young doctors, to get them caught up in taking care of a population that they may not wish to take care of.

I want them to begin to grapple with some of the basic questions of AIDS care: What am I doing here? What am I going to say to this man who is losing his lover? What am I going to say to this man who is a prisoner with a death sentence to begin with and now has AIDS? How can I give him emotional support? What do I say to parents to console them after they lose a child? Now that I have children, I know that there is nothing you can say to parents that will make them feel good when they lose a child.

I've learned that there is no right answer for many of these questions. To be part of someone else's experience of living and dying is emotionally challenging. No one trained me for that. In the mid-1970s, we had a sexual education course in medical school, which was innovative for the times. We were supposed to become desensitized in order to be able to talk about all these things with patients. In retrospect, the goal of the class was absurd. We were all in our early twenties. What did we know? We didn't know anything about death, and we certainly didn't know anything to talk about sexually. Now I deal with these issues all the time. My medical school at least acknowledged that it was important to be trained. We had courses, but none of what I learned really helped me. I guess the challenge is learning on the job.

There is no book called How To Be A Mentsch. But it actually turns out to be very easy if you don't let the barriers stop you. If I let the fact that someone is a prisoner get in the way, if I let it get in the way that I'm not a gay man, or I'm not an intravenous drug user or a woman who had twenty partners, then I would never be just a person with them. That was a real hurdle.

Probably the most emotionally challenging issue for me was deciding to come back after my needlestick. I really don't want to die, and I don't want to be sick. I don't want to be emotionally sick every day, worrying that I might become infected.

I don't believe AIDS is like the plague. If our present situation were like the bubonic plague, when the doctors really did die, I'm not sure what I would do. I'm not saying "kill me." I'm saying that I want to take care of people, and the risk is a little risk. It's one I can live with. Maybe if the numbers change ... if they tell me that every time you get stuck by a needle, you're going to get AIDS, then I wouldn't do this. Some people think that if you do AIDS care, you must be very altruistic. But I'm not. I'm not going to do something if I believe I am really risking my life. I still have a selfish side for my family and me. I still want to make it to retirement.

My Family

I should feel more guilty that I don't have more time with my kids. When I spend a lot of time with families who are taking care of either their dying children or their dying parents, part of me feels guilty that I don't spend as much time with my own children.

When I get home, my priority is my children. Actually, I don't feel like I've lost anything. If I didn't have children and wasn't doing anything, I would feel much more that I had missed out on what's happening here. It's kind of comparing apples and oranges now, and I have chosen to go with my kids, who are apples, and one day I will get back to having a little more time for some of the other things that I particularly enjoy. It was a lot easier before children, and I don't think that applies just to AIDS care workers. Before kids, there was a lot more time. With kids, it's very hard to have that emotional time.

The kids know what I do even though they are very little. They come up and see patients. I bring my children here. My family is not very happy that I have done that, but I feel that it's part of my life. They need to see what I do. They have gotten to know some of my patients. When patients call me at home, my kids are aware that someone is sick. I don't think I should make up a little fantasy for my kids about my job just because they're children.

I tell my children that I take care of people and help to make their lives a little bit better, but that many of them will die. Death wasn't a very real concept for my kids until recently when my father died. They are aware that when I can't be at home all day, I'm helping people who are sick. That makes me feel good. At least they know that I'm not getting my nails done and going shopping or something. I have overheard them telling their friends that their mommy takes care of very sick people.

I may be in therapy thirty years from now if it comes out that they couldn't stand that I did this. My parents and my in-laws met some of my patients and were in deep depression afterwards. They couldn't believe it. They kept saying, "How do you do this?" and "Why do you do this?" They still ask me why I don't go back into pediatrics. I never was in pediatrics. I just laugh. They have this idea that I should go back and do something I never did! Something happy. They're simply overwhelmed.

Risks and Fears

A lot of people think health care workers are particularly at risk and that it's very dangerous. I push that in the background because I don't think that it's particularly dangerous. For many of us who worked in New York and San Francisco in the early days of the epidemic, the risk of health care workers getting AIDS was not in the forefront of our minds. In our innocence, we probably jeopardized ourselves more than we care to think.

There are different levels of fear. For the first seven-and-a-half years of my AIDS work, I primarily took care of middle-class gay men. I was struck by the tremendous loss of creative young people to society. The last three-and-a-half years in public health, I primarily care for intravenous drug users, including prisoners. My initial sense of risk was really a fear of the prison population potentially hurting me.

Although I've always been treated with tremendous respect in the hospital setting, I realize that these prisoners probably wouldn't treat me with the same respect if I met them on the street. In recent years, I've been more fearful of who my patients are — not the fact that they have AIDS, but the crime and drug use that brought them to having AIDS. Lately, I've come to a very good balance. When people are sick, it really doesn't make any difference whether they are an upper-class theatrical producer or a poor man in prison for a crime. All the same fears and concerns are there.

My fears of needle risks to myself have very much increased over the past three years. I sustained a very serious needlestick a year ago and had to go on AZT. Doing this work, I always have to acknowledge that there is a risk. We constantly take precautions and continually talk to patients about safe lifestyles, safe sex, safe this, safe that. I give lectures on safety to health care workers, and every time I draw blood, I'm very aware of the risk. Even though I know that, statistically, the numbers are so much against anything happening, I wondered how I could have put myself and my children and husband at risk.

That needlestick shook me into active decision-making. I really had to think about why I do this work. It no longer worked for me to allow my passive choices based on the facts that I was good at doing this and had committed all of these years. It finally became a true active choice.

Fanning the Flames of Burnout

There is a risk that I'll become too burned out and too tired to really take care of myself. A lot of people get burned out whether it be cancer care, AIDS care, or other care. Maybe if and when the risk becomes greater, I'll leave AIDS work.

Last year when I had the needlestick, I had to put into better balance why I do this. I had to confront my family and ask them how they really felt about what I was doing. My husband, who was always somewhat unsupportive of what I did, finally acknowledged that I was good at what I did and that I got satisfaction from it. He didn't completely understand why I got as much satisfaction but told me that he would be more supportive, as long as the needlestick risk was as low as it really is.

Although I could never say that the needlestick was a good thing to have happened, it did make me crystallize a little bit more why I do what I do. It also made my family and friends confront what I do in a much more real way.

In order to take care of AIDS patients, you have to try to put the idea of personal risk in the background, even though it really is on the front burner all the time. While you're taking care of people and dealing with their issues every day, you can't constantly be worrying about the risk to yourself. You have to keep it tucked away or a very simple procedure may result in a great risk. It's a balancing act. People who really fear taking care of AIDS patients could probably never tuck it away. They couldn't push it to the background and still pay attention to it.

Working in the public health environment or any place in the United States where there are major budget cuts adds additional stress. We're asked to do more than our counterparts who work in institutions that have tremendous money and support. Even though I'm given a lot of credit, and people tell me it's wonderful what I do, it's very hard to be in an environment where after you plan programs, the programs are put on freeze. It's very hard to know that some people you work with and have helped train will lose their jobs.

When I came here three years ago, an assessment was done that showed us to be understaffed. Since then, we haven't had any additional staff, and all we've had is exponential growth of patients. Yes, I think I will burn out. I feel burned out many days. I feel burned out in advocating for prisoners' health care rights.

It's not a glitzy issue. People who aren't going to pay more taxes for their own children to go to school are certainly not going to pay more taxes for better health care for the mentally ill or prisoners with AIDS — the very areas that public health serves. So why am I knocking my head against the wall?

If someone recommends that I take time off, there's no one to cover for me. You can't really take time off because then there's no one to take care of your patients. You feel guilty if someone is dying, and you are not there.

After two or three years of taking care of someone, it's ironic when the one day you take off is the day they die. I've gotten much better when I'm on vacation, at being on vacation. I really don't want to be bothered. I think about what's going on, but I try very hard to let go of it. When I come home at night, I really am much better at letting go of it.

People acknowledge that hands-on AIDS caregivers are stressed out, but amid all the budget constraints and cuts and realities of the world, no one is really helping. People make a lot of recommendations, but nothing concrete happens after the recommendations.

I don't think I will still be doing what I do full-time twenty years from now. I wonder what I will do when I grow up. I'm grown up now, but I don't know if I can continue to take care of this population in this environment without additional, concrete help — not a "next year, we hope to possibly … if the budget gets better."

My day at the cancer center is a lot easier. There's a lot of stress with cancer work, but it's a beautiful environment. The concept of people being laid off is not quite as real. There's nice art work on the walls. There's the big foundation behind us. There's just an umbrella of positive feelings. It's not that anyone there covers for you when you're sick, but the environment is more supportive. At the cancer facility, where it's nice for middle-class gay men, and there is this beautiful hospital with many secretaries, it's a very different environment than in many AIDS settings. You don't get the sense that the world is about to end because of budget cuts.

You can get caught up in the sadness. That's the first focus of my family and friends. They say that it's too sad, or there are too many frustrations. I lost my father six weeks ago, and again, I face the reality of life being pretty short. I see it every day, and now, it hits me at home, too. My father died very quickly, and it was totally unexpected. I felt very angry at all my patients, both my cancer and my AIDS patients. They have so much more time to prepare and so do their families. Both my husband and I are in the field of medicine, and I think we really felt the irony of what we do. In our days of preparing patients and their families, we had no time to prepare for the death in our family. That was when I felt particularly burned out.

AIDS care is always very challenging emotionally, not just medically. Actually, the medicine part is probably the least provocative because I don't do lab research. I do clinical research. The lab scientists have a very different perspective of AIDS care. They are equally important to what we do, and they are the ones that will, I hope, bring us to a better state of medical care. But they are very removed from the scene. In the lab, there's a positive side. They do research, present a paper, get a name, and get credit, and it goes on their curriculum vitae. It looks very good. I've had that. You don't get to see someone dying, and that's a good side, too. But you don't get to see some of the positive things like patients who really do rejoin life. They're not all bogged down. A lot of us are more bogged down than the patients are.

A Ship Came In, A Ship Went Out: Feeling Ineffective

Even though I talk about this battle for quality of life, a lot of my patients are homeless and have no families. A team of us has brought a measure of comfort to their lives. When they die alone, there's no one to bury them and no one to acknowledge their lives and deaths. It's pretty crude, but you have to put an advertisement in the paper to see if anyone will claim the body. Even though we all helped make a difference, I feel very frustrated. No one even knows who this person was. A ship came in, and a ship went out. No one knew about it, and I wonder what the point is. What was all that energy I put into somebody that no one even knew or cared about other than us? I know that we cared about them. My God, these people just slipped in and out of life. Why did I miss my son in his kindergarten play? Why did I do this for a person who no one even knew? What was the point? That's when I feel ineffective.

I don't feel ineffective when someone dies. I really don't. I feel ineffective if someone didn't live, if they weren't able to do something from the time they met me. If they said they wanted to go visit their parents or whatever, and I couldn't mobilize them. When I mobilize them and get them onto medication, when I get them onto experimental protocols, I always feel good. If they die, that's just part of this disease. People are dying. People die from cancer. When I realize that there is nothing else to be done, I feel a sadness that we haven't yet made the stride. We haven't made that jump to the next drug. But I don't feel ineffective personally. Science today has made tremendous jumps from when I started taking care of AIDS patients in the early 1980s in New York. There are times when people die very quickly before we know what's happening, and I ask, "What could we have done?" That's natural in medicine. It's not unique to AIDS.

Feeling Effective, Being Effective

A lot of people who don't take care of AIDS or cancer patients think there's nothing else that can be done. They kind of give up the second the person walks in the door. I was consulted on a case where the team basically said, "Oh, he has AIDS. He's going to die, and there's no reason to do anything." I said, "You're wrong. There's a lot of very good treatment." I recommended that they do specific things, and the patient lived. He left the hospital and has been my patient for two years. Others were giving up on him, and my intervention helped.

I've worked very hard for two years to get the state to change its policy on prisoners who have AIDS. There was a policy in the state that if a prisoner was diagnosed with AIDS, he was quarantined in the hospital for the rest of his life. I was appalled by this because it made no medical sense. Prisoners should not be isolated based on a diagnosis. They were big, strapping, healthy men after I gave them treatment, and it was absurd that they were being locked on hospital wards for one, two, three years. They were not even allowed to go play basketball.

I know that this is a bleeding-heart-liberal issue, but I felt that this represented a human rights and an AIDS rights issue because people had a misconception about AIDS. They had a misconception about what health care is, and I was a thorn in the side of the correctional system. People told me not to do it, but I guess I was the new kid on the block coming to public health. I became a constant committee person attending various government meetings. I spoke, I testified, and I arranged educational programs. When the AIDS patients were allowed back into the general prison population, I felt very good. It was ironic that I got people to go back to prison, but that's what they wanted and that was the right thing. They were able to return to training programs and taking college courses, watching television and taking walks. I'm not an advocate for all prisoners, but I was an advocate that people with this disease should have human rights. I effectively spoke out and felt good about that.

Every time I meet with someone, a family member, a friend, or a lover who is afraid of this disease and afraid to embrace their loved one or not-so-loved one, I hold the person with AIDS to show how to be good to someone who is dying. I know when they hear from the nurses or social workers that it's okay, they take it in. When they hear the doctor say that it's all right to hug and touch, it's like I'm giving them a blessing. After I talk with someone, I always feel good when I see that person go into the room, remove the mask, and be able to be with someone who is sick — to let go a little bit of fear of touching and holding someone who has AIDS and may be dying.

In 1982, I helped take care of one of the first women in New York who had AIDS. In retrospect, it's so obvious that she had AIDS, but it wasn't obvious in the early 1980s. She was an intravenous drug user, and I was her resident and a big advocate for getting everything done for her. I was her only advocate. She had no family. I was struck by the fact that no one seemed to advocate for people who were all by themselves, the poor people, the nameless people who die.

I tracked people down and found her child. Although her condition turned out to be AIDS, and she ended up dying, it was a big step in my being a doctor and an advocate for patients. I still remember that, about a week before she died, she read this *Newsweek* article, the first big spread on this disease called AIDS. I explained to her that that was probably what she had, but very few women had the disease. At that time, they had no treatments, and it was so weird — we didn't wear gloves. We didn't do any of the little things that we do now.

This is the whole irony of people who took care of AIDS patients from 1980 through 1984. No one wore gloves. All of us who worked in New York and San Francisco were blissfully unaware of the risks. We knew there was some risk, but since we weren't having sex with the patients, we thought we were safe. I remember holding her hands. Her hands were covered with blood because she had these open wounds and, oh God....

Maintaining Sanity and Other Helpful Thoughts

I have two little kids, one is four and one is five. I'm burned out because I have two little kids. When I come home, I play with my kids. I watch *Jeopardy* every night. I like art and antiquing. I do that with my kids, but my kids don't exactly share my enthusiasm. I just spend more time with my family. Before I had children, I was much better at escaping. I really enjoy ballet. I would take a class, and I would regularly go to the ballet in New York and Washington.

I am also active in a community charity organization. It's a nice relief to help promote the mission of the organization, and I feel very good about doing something not medical and away from AIDS.

I'm very active in AIDS things in town. Within the last year or so, I have actually tried hard not to do that in my free time. It was an act of choice. I deal with AIDS every day. I can't make my whole life the world of AIDS.

I spend time with my children, husband, and family. I'm so exhausted after a whole day that I'm very happy to take a shower, read stories to my children, read a book, go through art magazines and antique journals. I do a lot of talking about doing things since I've had kids, but my husband is much better at the actual execution of these things. He's very good. He goes to the health club and works out every night, and he plays tennis. This is what I feel my colleagues and I should do, but I don't do it. I'm just extremely tired after I come home. I'm not good at saying, "This is my time," but I view it as my time with the kids.

The Media and Innocence vs. Guilt

People want to cubbyhole this disease. By separating themselves, it allows them to have some group of

people that they don't have to worry about. We don't have
to worry about those people. They did this to themselves.
But I resent that.

There are many people who are unaware that they
are at risk. There are other people who are aware that they
are at risk and who get this disease. I take care of many
intravenous drug users. They know all about AIDS, but they
have an illness called drug addiction that far surpasses their
ability to make a decision about getting AIDS. Even though
they can answer all the questions, their ability to translate
that into their lives is lost because they have another
disease.

The issues of AIDS and innocence and guilt are
bigger issues because people really have to grapple with
the issues of society and the disease of addiction. People
still view the addict as guilty. Almost all my patients are
innocent victims of this disease even though they may be
intravenous drug users or gay men or bisexual people or
prostitutes. The majority of the women I take care of have
been very sexually promiscuous because of their drug-use
history. But I personally never view them as anything but
innocent. I don't think anyone actively says, "I want
AIDS." The little baby with AIDS is much more eye-
catching — the innocent victim. I resent the fact that the
media use this to sell papers. It's good and bad. It's very
sad. It's a lot more chichi to raise money for a little baby
with AIDS or a movie star's wife who gets infected through
a blood transfusion. Half of my patients are what the media
would describe as the not-so-innocent victims. I take care
of a lot of prisoners with AIDS. I never want to know what
they're in prison for.

The media made this disease what it is. When it is
no longer chichi because the people who have it are not the

people that they think are worthy of front-page news, then it will be a back-page disease — like African AIDS.

Sexual Preference

I don't think my sexual preference has made a difference in my work. I am heterosexual, and I never entertained the thought of being a lesbian. My first boyfriend would have a good laugh now because I was pretty sexually repressed and not so liberal growing up in the 1960s and 1970s. If people who knew me then knew that I explain safe sex to white, black, and Hispanic men and talk about sexual preference with gay men, I think they'd have a good laugh. If they had to vote on what I would most likely not be talking about out loud to a group of people, it would certainly be that. I still laugh.

I don't pass judgment on someone who isn't heterosexual. As a woman, there's a certain sadness for me when I meet women who have been prostitutes. Just the thought that they've had to use their bodies that way makes me sad as a woman, and it has nothing to do with being heterosexual.

Some of the women are lesbian prostitutes, and some of the men that I have taken care of are gay prostitutes. I feel a certain sadness about the cavalierness of sex because I was never that cavalier. I don't view it as good or bad. It's just so different from the way I lead my own life.

I've been struck by the love that people have for each other regardless of their sexual preference. In that way, it has been a privilege to do AIDS work. Before, I never saw that side of the world. It's so sad that AIDS had to open up that part of the world to me. I'm now a big advocate for what goes on between two consenting adults behind closed doors.

The Privilege and the Challenge Continue

I got my gloves on and got into the fray. I didn't stand idly by. I feel good that it was a gift that was given to me to help people, and I did it. When I go through the numbers of patients that I have taken care of — hundreds of people who have died and probably more than a thousand that I have taken care of — that's very eerie to me. But I took care of them, and I thank them. I know that sounds silly to say, but it really was a privilege. It would have been a better privilege, perhaps, if I had had a magic pill to make everyone better, but I didn't, and I don't feel guilty about that.

I think the challenge in the future will really be a challenge to society, and it's going to be out of doctors' hands. I'm sure that we'll come up with a cure, but the real challenge to health care, of which AIDS care is a big part, is whether our country wishes to really embrace all the other problems. If people get burned out, the next batch of AIDS doctors who take care of the next part of the epidemic, will deal with the minority and poorer underbelly of the country. It's not a matter of giving out medications anymore. That's easy. It's giving out a house, giving out food, giving out day care for the child whose parents are sick, and giving out support for the grandparents who will take care of the child for the parents who are sick.

The greatest irony to me is that I now have all these medicines like AZT and Pentamidine in my "little black bag," but I don't have what else it's going to take to help someone have a good life. Many of my patients don't have a house or someone to take care of their kids. Their husband is in prison or is on the street. They are sexually abused. The AIDS part is easy. I can give them medicine, but the rest is what's boggling.

Chapter Four

Elaine: Amidst the Frequency of Decline and Death

It's sadder for me because I get to know people over a longer period and learn their stories. You don't forget their stories.

A physical therapist for eleven years, Elaine has worked with people with AIDS for one-and-a-half years, fifteen in the last twelve months, in a rehabilitation unit within an acute hospital. She is a thirty-two-year-old white, heterosexual woman, who is newly married. Her high energy and enthusiasm for her work burst out during our visit.

Elaine feels lucky to be the physical therapist in the case management group, soaking up information from colleagues who have worked with AIDS patients longer. She's learning to deal with aspects of the disease so that she can better help her patients cope with what's going on in their lives.

Even though she was raised "extremely Catholic," she has parted company with organized religion. Judgmental perspectives on people and their behavior don't work well for her with the patients she treats. She believes that she is much more open-minded and accepting of differences among people.

With all the uncertainty and ups and downs of AIDS, she feels like she's constantly riding a roller coaster.

Empowerment and Gratification

Working with this patient population is very empowering for me as a therapist. It engages and challenges me on so many different levels. I work with other patients besides, but with my AIDS patients I feel much stronger in my patient communication and my ability to really get down to the point at hand. As I continue the work, I'm not as afraid of the glitches that you run into — the family members who are worked up about something or the patient who's really struggling with something. It has helped empower me to be stronger clinically and personally, to work through my anxieties or check them at the door. When I am connecting with the patient, I'm more able to focus all my energy rather than having it dissipated into my own anxieties about this and that. My growth has to do with focus, channeling my therapeutic energies, and being there for all patients, not just those with AIDS.

I've been very moved by people with AIDS. It's so gratifying. We all went to the AIDS Committee annual awards dinner where one of our doctors in the AIDS clinic was getting an award. I was new and didn't think I should be a part of it. There were hundreds of people all doing this kind of work. It was mind-boggling! I was so impressed!

What do I do with this? I'm still learning a lot and feeling like I need to bring myself up to speed, even if only on a purely academic level. I need a good understanding of the disease process. It's also satisfying on an intellectual level because I'm reading and doing and reading some more. I feel very stimulated by this information. I don't know where this is going to lead me. Loss of functional mobility is a major problem with AIDS, and the patients need strong role models in physical therapy. I don't yet know how I'll take it from here. This is a huge area for expansion in our profession. Strong clinicians and communicators are needed to help the patients with their plans and help them with their decision making.

Sexual Preferences — The Patients' and My Own

I don't feel that my sexual preference has made a difference in my work. Nobody has asked me about my sexual preference. Both of the women I've treated were bisexual. Not the men. I've never thought that this would be easier for me if I were homosexual or bisexual. I haven't felt that it has gotten in the way or that I've been shut out because people assume that I am or appear to be heterosexual or that I mention my husband. In my life, I've had real interactions and personal relationships with male and female homosexuals. That probably has put me in a different place than some of the other therapists I've worked with who just don't get it. Sexuality is just a fact.

It's not just a matter of my preference. If patients thought I had negative feelings about their preference, I would feel like I had shot myself in the foot therapeutically. Patients sense these things. They know. If I had issues with it, at a conscious or subconscious level, they would come across somehow. I wouldn't be able to do what I do as effectively if my patients felt that I couldn't relate or be there for them because I don't share their particular preference.

Clinical and Other Challenges

There are several levels to working with people with AIDS. The more work I do, the more levels become apparent. When I first targeted this patient population, I was doing it purely from a clinical point of view. Looking at the literature, I realized that there was a wealth of information and body of patients, and I was very interested in how the people with AIDS were presenting from a neurological point of view. On a clinical level, it's exciting that there's a lot of information available, with new information being generated all the time.

People with AIDS are intellectually challenging to work with because they have the neurological symptoms I'm used to seeing as a physical therapist, but the reasons are not as clear. It's also exciting clinically because of the multi-system involvement of the patients. I've been a clinician working in acute settings for many years, but now I need to integrate a lot of information to treat one person.

I don't think that clinicians can completely separate their personal and professional selves. Although I've worked in different settings with a variety of patients and have experienced the death of some of my patients, I've never had a patient population for which dying was the typical course of events. Watching patients "crump" before my eyes is very difficult, especially when it's a number of patients, not just one or two, who I know will decline.

On a personal level, I struggle with the real sorrow of watching my patients go downhill. As with other patients, I get to know them as people. I meet their friends, families, lovers, support people — all those people who are struggling with the same kind of loss. I may be sadder because this patient population is still fairly new to me. Each time there is a death or somebody "bottoms out," I experience that at a "whammo" level. I've asked the social worker on the AIDS team, "How the hell have you been doing this for years? How do you do it? How do you take care of yourself? Do you ever get yourself to the point you're not wrecked for a couple of days every time this happens?" We talked about coping, which I think will be an ongoing struggle.

Some of the physicians I work with have run AIDS clinics for years and have followed some patients for that whole time. When a patient declines and/or dies, they still take it very much to heart. I don't think it's just a matter of time and experience. If I'm doing this work three years from now, I don't know that I'll be coping any better. I'll probably need to figure out how to take care of myself given the certain inevitability that a number of patients who I'm involved with over a long period of time, will die. My job is both a drag and exciting at the same time. Sometimes, I wonder why the hell I am doing this. What am I doing with this patient population? At a very human level, it's hard to be around all the sorrow.

At a professional level, the dynamic of treating these patients is challenging. There's not a whole lot of help out

there for physical therapists who are coming into contact
with these patients. Certainly no one is targeting this population. Even though there is more information now showing
up in our professional literature about how to deal with this
patient population, I find that I turn to other health professionals — social workers, nurses, physicians — for help
with other issues. I have some ideas about how I would like
to see our profession address this tremendously needy
population. There's a real role for physical therapy here, yet
we've barely scratched the surface.

The biggest challenge for me is trying to be there for
patients at the end stage of their disease, when they're struggling with issues of mortality, AIDS, and losses. In trying to
be present for them, I need to integrate all the available
information. I struggle to form and maintain consistently
effective relationships. This decline of patients doesn't
come along once in a blue moon with AIDS, and my biggest
challenge is trying not to be overwhelmed.

Learning from The Emir

During the Gulf War, I worked with a man I called
"The Emir." His name sounded like those on the news every
night, and he agreed that this nickname was a good compro-
mise for an otherwise long name. He was not quite forty
years old, a black gentleman whose risk factor for AIDS was
his homosexuality. When I started in the AIDS case-manage-
ment group, I first heard about him during rounds. He was
very ill with just about every AIDS-defining illness in the
book. He would come in with PCP (pneumocystis carinii
pneumonia) and then lymphoma. They gave him a shot, his
lymphoma improved markedly, and then he "crumped"

again. He amazingly bounced back from a very life-threatening stage, and I was asked to evaluate him. Everyone was amazed that he was going to be leaving the hospital.

When I met him, I thought he was probably the tallest, skinniest guy I had ever met. He was six feet tall and used to dance ballet. He was a practicing Buddhist, which was also new to me. At that point, he was very motorically impaired, had terrible peripheral neuropathy, and poor mobility. Bed-to-chair movement was the most he was doing. After his courses of chemotherapy, he wasn't eating much and had lost a tremendous amount of weight.

Over the weeks that we worked together, he got his appetite back and was starving all the time. I had never seen such a skinny man eat so much. He would hoard food all the time. I swear he was stealing it from other people's trays. One day, he was complaining about being hungry, and I made the big mistake of giving him something to eat. We'd had a party in the morning, and there were some bagels left over. The next day, when he came for exercise he looked at me and said, "What, no bagels? No bagels, no exercise. If I'm going to do all this work, I want to be fed." It was the funniest thing — here was this "Mr. No Bagels, No Exercise," with a nickname of "Emir." I, of course, bought into this entitlement and would bring him food. People in the department had no idea what was going on. This tall, totally wild-looking man would be lounging on the mat table, licking his fingertips and wiping the cream cheese off the corner of his mouth. He reached a point of ambulating a few hundred feet and was really making some gains. When he left to go to another facility, we gave him food as a going-away present.

Through the grapevine, I kept updated on how he was doing, and we'd send regards to each other. Just when we were going to connect again, I heard that he was having more problems with his gait and falling down the stairs. It was decided that it was a recurrence of his lymphoma. Within the course of a week and a half, he went into a hospice and died.

The Emir struck me for a few reasons. He was the first person I treated in this patient population who wasn't an IV drug abuser. He was the first person I became close to who didn't have the behavioral issues that I saw with people who were substance abusers. The majority, if not all, of the patients I'd had up to that time, had been actively abusing a substance and themselves for years. The Emir was the first man I treated whose risk factor was homosexuality. He talked openly about being gay and having AIDS. He had seroconverted and had his first AIDS-defining illness years ago. He had already processed so much, and I was learning from him.

As a Buddhist, he strongly believed that he was going to come back again to work through whatever he hadn't worked through in this life. I remember his views on dying and death, which were so different from those patients with a Western point of view. He used to give me his Buddhist newspapers to read and would meditate in his room. I heard that he raised a ruckus one night when his Buddhist meditation group came in to meditate with him. Apparently the chanting caused quite an uproar on the floor. More power to him!

Shattering Illusions

When I came to this downtown hospital, with its big population of people who are homeless, drug abusing, sort of rough-neck-of-the-woods, it was very different from the small community hospitals where I had worked. This place certainly gave me a much wider exposure to people who were HIV-positive and people who had big risk factors. It has only been in the last year and a half that I've targeted the AIDS population.

One of my dearest friends is a gay man, and I've been exposed to the male gay population over a period of time. I didn't have a hard time with people's sexuality and thought that homosexuality was an issue that I already knew. There's so much inherent bigotry against people with AIDS, as though they deserve to have it. Some of the first HIV people I treated in this facility were women who were substance abusers.

I treated a young, heterosexual woman in another facility where there hadn't ever been a person with AIDS. She was very unclear about why she had AIDS. She shattered every illusion I had about people with AIDS being homosexual men, IV drug abusers, or someone whose lifestyle would somehow link them up with this disease. At that point, I think I erased whatever undercurrent of bigotry I was carrying around in my own heart. Here was a young woman who was about my age, in her early twenties. Her husband was not HIV-positive. She had been healthy up to that point and came into the hospital with PCP. The diagnosis of AIDS was made.

Here was a young, professional woman with a few sexual partners in the past, certainly nothing that anybody would label as promiscuous. It was unclear as to when and why this happened, but there it was. That was a big struggle for me as a PT, as a person, and as a woman. That gave me a unique opportunity to take a very hard look at myself and really come to terms with some of my beliefs about people with this illness. It has helped me to another point of consciousness in being able to treat AIDS patients more effectively.

Guilt, Innocence, and Avoidance

I hear about the guilty and innocent issue all the time because it runs rampant in the presentation of AIDS and the public understanding of people with AIDS. They think that AIDS is something that homosexuals, prostitutes, or people who abuse drugs get. The Ryan Whites of the world and the hemophiliacs are a whole different animal and somehow deserve compassion and an outpouring of support that these other people don't deserve. Because AIDS is a social issue, and anybody working in a hospital setting is part of the social world, there are no guarantees that a caregiver is a person who doesn't carry a negative viewpoint.

When I first targeted the AIDS population, I told a doctor on the infectious disease service that I wanted to see anybody with motoric kinds of signs. At the time, the infectious disease service was filled with people who were difficult to manage behaviorally, such as some active IV drug abusers, who were always causing a ruckus and threatening to sign out. I will never forget one person who looked me right in the eye and said, "Why would you ever want to do that? Why would you want to do this at all?" It stuck with me.

On one hand, people in my own department wonder why I would be interested in this patient population. On the other hand, at some level they're glad that I'm doing it because it means that they don't have to. It's a scary thing because you can't work with AIDS patients and not come up against your own fears about having the disease transmitted to you. Many caregivers struggle to form an effective therapeutic relationship with patients who they might feel, somewhere deep down, really deserve to have AIDS and don't deserve their full effort as a therapist. By my getting involved in AIDS care, I let some other people off the hook.

A few times, I had face-to-face encounters with other therapists who point blank refused to cover a patient for me when I was on vacation. What do you do when somebody doesn't want to be in a room, even though it's a professional expectation? When I came to work here, I asked colleagues how they felt about treating people with AIDS, those with HIV infection, or heroin abusers without known infection yet who were shooting up two days ago in the streets. I got nothing but, "We're good, we're fine." But when individual cases came up, some of the therapists had a lot of feelings about it, a lot of nervousness, a lot of angst about seeing these people.

At this facility, we see more and more children born with AIDS, and people seem to put them in the "innocent" category — AIDS was something that was done to them; they didn't do anything to deserve this, unlike their parents.

I've asked how health workers feel about having to be physically close to people with AIDS, but I don't feel the issue has been addressed. I don't feel that I could have a forum here, or at any place else I work, for a really honest discussion of how individuals feel about treating people with AIDS. I believe that there are prejudices and fears. I don't expect that physical therapists, nurses, doctors, or other health workers feel differently than anyone else. They come to work with their backgrounds, thoughts, families, upbringing, views on society, and ideas of how we all fit into it. It's a hard topic to bring up and discuss.

I think there's an assumption that in order for physical therapists to work with AIDS patients, they have to be absolutely fine with it — that one conflicting emotion or thought is seen as a failing. If they voiced their concerns, they would be less of a professional, less of a caregiver. All of the emotion keeps getting buried.

When I go over universal precautions with staff and students, it makes my heart rate go up. When you read it, it's the real stuff. Despite their angst and avoidance behavior, they're not admitting, "I don't want to go into those rooms. Look at all the stuff I have to do just to touch that patient or not touch them."

Fear and Comfort

I haven't felt afraid of physical transmission to myself. Some patients have a lot of problems with skin breakdown and general drainage from Kaposi's sarcoma, but I feel very comfortable with that. I take care of myself and feel comfortable with gowning and gloving and doing anything I need to do here. I do a fair amount of work in the intensive care units so I'm around people who have precautions for different reasons. To me, this is just another precaution to take.

Other people, though, get anxious. I hear people say, "When I told my husband, boyfriend, or my father, or whoever, that I'm treating someone with AIDS, I got this big response." I haven't received any negative reaction, although my parents sometimes wonder what I'm doing. My brother, who is doing some AIDS research, said, "I knew you were going to work yourself around to this." He expressed some concern, but he was fine after we talked about it. I'm not sure where my husband is in all of this. He certainly knows that I do this and has never expressed any consternation. I'm glad I'm not getting negative pressure. I think that's what unnerves people the most.

When you're here and looking at yourself as a professional, you know what you need to do to have all your bases covered. It's different to go home every night and have people horrified. They want to make sure that you're safe. You can't get caught up in the fear that the general public has. That makes it harder.

Anxiety and Sorrow

My anxieties have to do with a person's overall emotional dynamic in the situation. When I first meet a patient, there is a certain amount of anxiety until I establish a rapport with them. I typically meet people who are further along in their disease process, and my anxieties are still there. I don't breezily go into any of these patients' rooms. I really stop and think about it and get myself where I need to be. That initial connection is so important in how I'm going to be read — how much is this person going to buy into seeing me, how I can establish myself as somebody who they can let back in, somebody positive in their lives.

Another component of my anxiety is dealing with homosexual lovers, the patient's significant other and their biggest support, as opposed to the wives, husbands, mothers, daughters, and sisters. Seeing how the rest of the patient's family reacts to the fact that he is gay or she is bisexual and has AIDS is intense. It's a relationship that I was not used to dealing with, and some of my anxieties centered around how I could be there for the patient.

I don't have a lot of experience with this kind of sexual relationship. Although I have dealt with family members who are angry at their loved ones dying, the added element here is that these families are sometimes angry because of the nature of the diagnosis. Suddenly, they're facing a whole dimension of the patient's life that may have been hidden away. I am an integral part of that dynamic because I'm making plans for people to go home and live. I also see my role in helping everybody else figure out what to do, particularly with issues around somebody going home, care and services needed, and help for walking. I feel anxious about trying to get that across and make sure everybody is getting what they need.

I can't recall feeling angry with some of the patients, even some of the patients with behavioral issues who have given all of us on the team a run for our money. I'm used to that. I've been a physical therapist long enough in acute care settings to understand that sometimes I'm the last person a patient wants to see coming through the door. As much as they might want to get back on their feet, the message is "not now."

When I'm working with patients who are making decisions about how aggressive they want their course of treatment to be, I feel a lot of anxiety and sorrow. I'm seeing people at the point when they're really coming to terms with the big picture, when they're weighing things like hospice versus going home again. They're dying and will die soon, and it's sad.

I remember a young woman whom I worked with for three-and-a-half months. She hadn't been out of the hospital in that whole time, and we finally got to the point where she was going home. On her first day home, she called me, crying out of control. When she calmed down, she told me that the therapist from the Visiting Nurse Association (VNA) had put gloves on when she went to do her leg exercises. This was a woman with no lesions. She was totally continent in bowel and bladder. It just flipped her out because it was her first exposure to being perceived as unclean. God, what she was up against! I called the VNA, and they told me that using gloves was their policy, period.

I have a knee-jerk response to the age of the people that I'm seeing. They're so young. Although there's a lot of work going on with the disease, I see the progression. I treated a gentleman here, a homosexual, who had been well known to the rest of the AIDS team for years. I saw him really late in his course. He was a tremendously intellectual guy, working on his PhD in history. It meant so much to him to be able to finish it. He expired three days after I met him. We packed a big life story into those three days. His death devastated the social worker who had known him. Although he was a total mess, he still had a bit of hope that he could go home for a little while and finish his doctorate. But that didn't happen.

Since I've been in acute care, I haven't tracked a particular patient population over a long time, but I now end up reconnecting with people. In rehab, patients may be a mess, but physical therapists get them to a point to go home. They help them change how they feel and how they expect to lead their lives. There is a life in there somewhere. I know that at the end of all of this, there's a death in there. My sorrow with this population is the same as my sorrow with the oncology population that I see from time to time. Part of the sorrow is over any loss of life.

All-in-One:
Most Effective, Least Effective

I became a player in one life story and felt the most effective and least effective in the same situation. In my early days, I treated a woman who was an IV drug abuser reaching the end stage of her disease. She yelled and swore a lot and was just wild. She presented like someone with paraplegia and needed quite a bit of heavy musculoskeletal work. Whenever I came into her room, she cursed like a mule driver at me. That was part of my least effective interaction. I let her agenda get in my way and was frightened by her obnoxiousness, by the fact that she was young and neurologically "crumping." I had never seen anybody who had taken a dive so fast. A month earlier, she was walking around and then she fell apart.

I felt I needed to protect her somehow, but she was just right there in my face. She would yell at me, "Why in the hell should I let you come in here and do this stuff with me? I'm going to die you know. I'm going to die from AIDS. Don't you know I have AIDS? Why are you doing it?" I got so flustered that I would have to leave and come back. I would think about it overnight. That was the point where I initially felt the least effective because I had such a hard time being there. She asked very valid questions. There was no reason for her to put up with me coming in to stretch her painful, spastic legs and teach her how to transfer to a wheelchair. She was going to die and probably soon. I hung in there, though, for whatever reason. She was there, and I needed to be doing something with her.

One day, before the hospital went smoke-free, I took her to the smoking area so she could have a cigarette. It was actually a bribe. Since she couldn't smoke in her room, if she got into her wheelchair and maneuvered it to the smoking area, she could get rewarded. She said, "I can stay here for a while." The room was packed with other people chatting and smoking. I went to do something else and came back to get her. What had been a full room of people now looked like someone had pulled the fire alarm — everybody had taken off, and there was my patient sitting in the middle, smoking her cigarette.

Knowing she was not particularly inhibited, I asked her where everyone went. She said, "I guess they got a little nervous when I told them I had AIDS," and she burst out laughing. We sat there, and I laughed till I cried because I could just picture her. She laughed, "Now I have all the ashtrays."

It helped move me along. I wasn't quite as overt as people in the smoking area who got up and left, but I had been getting up and leaving her a little bit every day. That experience propelled me into being with her all the way. She continued to "crump," and things didn't change that much. We still fought, and I still bribed her. It was still kind of a mess of a treatment, but I felt that my effectiveness was better because she couldn't scare me away anymore.

Team Support Keeps Me Going

I'm always asking the social worker, "How do you take care of yourself when all this happens?" I need to be continually reminded that I need to take care of myself. I'm in the enviable position that I have a mixed-bag job description and patient load. If I feel overwhelmed, such as when I had all AIDS patients who were dying at the same time, I can call the social worker or go to AIDS rounds and talk about how I'm feeling. I like the support group because you can be vocal or remote and have it be okay. I can say, "I don't know how everybody else is doing with this, but I'm totally and completely sad around these people." Of course, some of them might say, "Not all this sorrow again, get the hook, get her out of here." But you can see that other people are sad, too, because it's a sad thing. I feel lucky that there are people around. I don't feel like I'm the only person who is struggling with this whole human and emotional thing.

People cry. The attending physicians cry. People are totally distressed and overwhelmed and exhausted, so it helps to be in that setting. I feel I can always go there.

If I didn't have these people here who I can connect with, I don't think I'd ever be able to target this patient population, even though I find them clinically fascinating. I need support and to share insights with others who have also chosen to treat these people. There is a role here for us, but I wouldn't be able to do it without these people.

Spirituality

I was raised Catholic, but I haven't been practicing under the auspices of the church for a number of years. I don't think that working with people with AIDS has driven me back to or away from the church, but it has given me a lot more to contemplate. Although it hasn't changed the organized aspect of my religious practices, it probably has made me let go of some of my issues around fairness and unfairness. I agree more with that bumper sticker, "Shit Happens."

Working with people with AIDS, I've learned more about myself and my own spirituality as a constant process. I know I've grown as a person, but I can't put my finger on how. I've always thought about the growth and development of my own soul.

Having a Jesuit priest doing pastoral care as part of the AIDS team probably makes a difference. We know how the patients are walking, how their insurance is working out, how their infections are doing, but how are their souls? He gives us a spiritual update. I was amazed when I first heard him report to the team. Everyone, including the attending physicians, stopped and listened with total respect. Spirituality often gets lost in patient care. We tend to get a sense of how people are dealing with their disease on a purely emotional, day-to-day level. To see the patients place such spiritual value on issues around this illness is incredible to me. It's not making me go to Mass, however, so my mother would probably think that it doesn't count.

Chapter Five

Kim: Small Losses and Other Heartaches

*I've worked very hard trying to get out of here after
the end of my eight hours. I try really hard to leave this
place behind when I go home. I don't always succeed.*

Fifty-year old Kim is a heterosexual woman of
color. A nurse for six years, she has worked with AIDS
patients for three years and has treated more than 100 AIDS
patients in the past year in a long-term public hospital.

Although she's much older than many of the nurses
she works with, she has less nursing experience than many.
Her age makes her more like their mother, she says, but her
professional position has her learning from them. She's very
detail-oriented, something which is important on the job but
needs to be softened at home.

Kim and her husband of almost thirty years have
raised two children, now grown. Their daughter has been in
a monogamous relationship for four years, but their twenty-

five-year-old son is dating — out on the "open market" — a source of concern for Mom in this day of AIDS.

She believes that the white patients regard her as "exotic." They were accustomed to seeing white nurses at their bedside and "in strides this tall, black woman." Some of their comments strike her as reverse discrimination and are hard to take. Some of the patients of color also snub her, calling her an *Oreo,* black on the outside, white on the inside. This hurts even more.

It's less difficult for Kim to deal with the loss of life than it is for her to cope with the mental and physical deterioration that leads to death. Dealing with all of the small losses along the way exacts a tremendous toll.

On the Cutting Edge and Other Challenges

Being on the cutting edge of AIDS treatment and research was one of the reasons I chose to work with people with AIDS. When I started this, we were really on the cutting edge of all the AIDS therapies. I wanted to do something in medical-surgical nursing, but I wanted to do something unusual. Three years ago, most of the drugs we used weren't even in the PDR (Physicians' Desk Reference) or nursing handbooks. They were all study drugs that have now become FDA-approved. Today, they're common. Three years ago, we were turning people with AIDS away because we had only a ten-bed unit. Things have turned around. Hospices have opened, drugs are more well-known, visiting nurse services are widely used, and people are doing a lot more at home. A lot of AIDS patients can be maintained at home if they have a significant other and if their dementia is not too significant. We're entering a new phase.

Another reason I began working with AIDS patients was a sense of heroics. When I came to this unit, the majority of the patients were people of color, and they had no people of color working here in any professional capacity. There was one aide. When I did my nursing training, I took care of Caucasian patients mostly, in predominantly Caucasian hospitals. I think I was regarded as an oddity. If there was a black patient, I was always assigned to him. I felt that the delivery of health care to them was a little bit different. Most of them expressed to me some feeling of discomfort. I wanted to be in a place where I could help alleviate that in some way.

I'm challenged by working with AIDS patients and being in my new position. I'm still learning my job. I find myself going back to the role of being a staff nurse because I was very comfortable there. Here I'm responsible not only for the patient's well-being, but also keeping up with everything that's going on with the staff. Sometimes, I get focused on one group, and the other group slides. The patients set the tone. If we have a difficult patient for weeks at a time, the staff can dread getting up in the morning because they know what's facing them. It's always a challenge trying to keep the staff motivated, buoyed up, and still trying to do the best for the patients.

When I interview people to work on this unit, one of the first things I look for is what I call a bleeding-heart personality — somebody who is prepared to put AIDS patients in their graves, somebody with a hospice mentality. I don't encourage people to work on this unit who feel that people hospitalized with AIDS are ready to die. True, a lot of them are ready to die, but you don't want to go into a room with an attitude of pity. Inside, you have an abundance of feelings because here is a young person before you who should be in his or her prime. It doesn't matter how they got it, whether they got infected because they're a drug addict or gay or whether it's from heterosexual contact. You can't help feeling something and silently saying, "My God, your life is, in effect, over."

Knowing that there's no cure in the pipeline makes it very difficult. Dealing with AIDS isn't like dealing with cancer. If you have cancer, the first thing people say to you is, "I'm sorry about that," but they blame people with AIDS. "You got it. It's your fault." It's hard to keep blame out of your thinking. As a health professional, you should be able to, but we're people, too.

The Effectiveness–Ineffectiveness Continuum

I remember a patient who was here for over a year and a half. When she was admitted, she had sight problems and was medically difficult to manage because of multiple diagnoses. During her stay, she was stabilized through many conferences with all the health care personnel. Her family even saw her in a new light. They saw how she had been managed on this unit and realized that they would be able to take her home, which they did. In the back of our minds, we were saying, "We give that a week. We give that two weeks." It's been a while now, and the family calls us less often. This is a real success story. When she was admitted, we said that she would never go home because she's too difficult. We kept plugging along. The patient also got to know us better, and as she trusted us, her compliance increased. Our persistence paid off. More than a year and a half later, she got to go home.

There are a lot more times when I feel ineffective. We have a lot of drug abusers. I have difficulty with the young, black, male drug abusers, probably because I have a young, black son. When I look at people in that age group, one part of my mind says, "Thank God, that's not my child." The other part of me sometimes regards these guys as my children. This becomes highly personal for me. I wonder why they did this to themselves.

We had a young man in his early thirties who made his living on the streets, hustling or doing one illegal thing after another. A neuropsychiatric evaluation turned up a learning disability. I wondered if he could have been helped if his mother had known. He left school in the seventh grade. Could his life have been different? It's just a very frustrating feeling. Eventually, we helped the man to die well. He was one of the ones that went out kicking and screaming. He was never ready for hospice.

When I first came here, it was about eighteen months from diagnosis to death. People go for years now with the better medications so I think of trying to improve their lives — getting continuing care, encouraging them to go after public housing, or something like that. That makes me feel effective. When they get over this bout of pneumonia or that infection and leave here, they disregard all of your good advice. Then we hear that they've come into the outpatient clinic, and they've been out drugging. I think that I didn't do a very good job, but maybe it wasn't the job to do.

This Isn't the World I Made:
Feeling Helpless

I have to let go of thinking I can save the world. If somebody is addicted, he may not have come in here to do anything about his addiction. They come in because they have cellulitis or a flare-up of some illness, like PCP (pneumocystis carinii pneumonia). They didn't come in for you to help them with their drug addiction. They didn't come in for you to help them with their lives. Sometimes, I feel very nursely.

This isn't the world I made. He didn't ask me for help for this so I shouldn't blame myself for not being able to help him. If I'm not angry at myself, I'm angry at the patient, angry at the world, angry at the system. The system could have done better by this person. There are not enough programs out there. We can change some situations. Maybe we could make something better. It's not minor when you can get VNA assistance for somebody, and it's not minor if you can find housing, and it's not minor if you can gather all the forces together to find help. This is all you're going to be able to do. At times, I feel helpless.

AIDS is still a terminal disease and no matter what you do they're going to die. The hopeful part of it is that prevention is getting better, and a lot of the treatments are changing. They're giving steroids very early on to people with exacerbations of PCP, so that the lungs don't get inflamed and there's less destruction. They used to give high doses of AZT, which made a lot of people anemic and sick to their stomachs. Now, they're getting fairly decent results with lower doses. So there's more compliance. If you can marshal all your efforts and the patient is compliant, that's the hopeful part. They have a better quality of life. Some of the patients are very gung ho and are going to do absolutely everything to keep themselves healthy.

Anger, Anger, Anger

When I'm ill-treated by some of the patients, three things flash in my mind. The first thing is a gut-level, human response — somebody said something really rotten to me, and I want to get them back. The second part is, they have a right to say this because they have AIDS, and they're young and dying. The third thing is, wait a minute, even though they're young and dying, they don't have a right to abuse me like this. All these things go through my mind, ten and twelve times a day, with almost every interaction. When I get to know the patient, I sometimes take a little bit more abuse because I know the patient is having a bad day, and the next day he's going to say he's sorry. Having this disease or any other fatal disease does not necessarily make you into Nicky Nice Guy. If he was an SOB before he had AIDS, generally he's an SOB with AIDS.

As a nurse, I'm always writing up care plans. If the patients follow this, they can get better — not necessarily cured, but better. When somebody isn't compliant, we run into trouble. We ask sick people to do something that they don't want to do. Our jaws drop when our volunteers say, "Mr. So and So is such a nice person." I get nothing but grief from this man when I ask him anything. The difference, of course, is that the volunteer says, "Would you like to go for a walk?" "Can I take you outside?" "What can I bring you?" I say, "You're going to take this medicine that makes you sick," or "I'm going to have to do a painful procedure." What do you expect?

This is what I have to deal with sometimes. For my
own safety and sanity, I can't ignore this and take it all into
myself. Some staff members absorb all this stuff. They
never give any of their anger back to the patient or say,
"You can't abuse me like this. I'm here to help you, but you
can't get away with this." If you don't have the capacity to
do that, you're not going to last in this field very long. A lot
of people don't. They become a sponge, taking it all in, and
have no place to go with their feelings.

Every once in a while, there's a patient who strikes
a chord. There was a male transsexual who had lived for
two years as a female. He had been through the psychiatric
evaluation and was getting ready to have surgery when he
was discovered to be HIV-positive. Of course, that
cancelled everything. She — I always referred to her by her
female name even though she was still a man — reminded
me so much of my sister, I was absolutely devastated. I
could have put her on the phone with my mother, and my
mother wouldn't have known that this was not her other
daughter. Her mannerisms, style, absolutely everything
seemed like my sister. It was bizarre. She made such a
strong connection with me, I was drawn to this person.

I was very angry at this patient's family because
they were totally unaccepting of her way of life. When she
was buried, her significant other was completely shut out of
the funeral services and the burial. This person who had
dressed and presented herself as a woman for two years was
put into a suit of men's clothing and laid to rest that way. I
think that's totally inappropriate.

We see patients over years, and sometimes I get
attached to a patient. The patient–professional relationship
becomes a little bit blurred because I get involved with the
families a lot more. If there are no families, we often

become these people's significant others for decision making and discharge planning. They have nobody to talk to and will ask for our advice. They talk to us about everything. Sometimes, they're alienated from family and friends, and we get everything that a wife, lover, or friend would have gotten. At other times, we get a lot of their anger because they don't want to alienate their wives, lovers, or friends. That's one of the hazards of being a health care professional.

I always feel guilty about getting angry. If someone curses at me, calls me all sorts of foul names, threatens to hit me, I feel that I have a right to get angry. I'm only human. When I think about it later, I say to myself, "Thank God, it's not me. He's angry at me, but I'm going home after eight hours."

Occasional Sadness, Occasional Laughter

I feel sad on occasion. When I know a patient has fought particularly hard but is going to die, I feel sad. Sometimes, I feel relief. We have had people here who have undergone brain biopsies. This is absolutely staggering to me to allow somebody to do a brain biopsy when all they're going to say is, "Yes, you definitely have the disease." It's amazing that patients would allow it, but hope springs eternal.

Every once in a while, I get a really good laugh, and it's never planned. I'll just be talking to patients, and it doesn't become patient–nurse anymore. I hope they can let go of the fact, for a minute, that they have AIDS, but I don't see how it doesn't color every minute of their waking days.

Sometimes, I feel funny when I go in and ask them what movie do they want to see. I think, "God, that sounds like such a lame question. What do they care?" But they look at these things, they discuss it, they talk about the world situation just like anybody else.

Small Losses and Other Sorrows

The loss of life doesn't bother me as much anymore because it comes with the territory. The hurtful part is seeing people in the twenty to forty age range that are showing the deep dementia of an eighty-five-year-old. That's the most difficult part. That's a part that I have to recognize and get over with every patient. I'll be teaching a thirty-five-year-old man something, and he might not be getting it, either because of full-blown dementia or the start of short-term memory loss. I have to remind myself every time that this person isn't being recalcitrant. This person has some dementia, and I shouldn't expect too much. I have to see what level of functioning he's capable of and teach according to that level. Sometimes, the teaching needs to be very concrete and basic — the men's bathroom is down there, or this is your room.

A few times I've seen people slip so much. I knew them when they were well, and then they became demented and wandered. The first time I had to explain to an otherwise oriented high school teacher that I had to put a *Posey* vest on him to restrain him for his own safety, we both cried. He was unable to comply with calling the nurse when he wanted to get up and would fall every time. Putting him in a *Posey* killed me. That was one of the roughest things I ever did.

These day-to-day things are the difficult things. When they die, it's hard, but it's not that hard. It's not as hard as taking away cigarettes and matches from a twenty-eight-year-old and making him come to the desk or turn his light on when he wanted to smoke, so that he could be supervised. It's not as hard as having them lose control of their bladder and bowels. This is real sad. It's hard for us because we're talking to an otherwise competent patient about *Depends,* saying, "Are you going out? Do you have enough diapers with you?" Or they'll be talking to you and say, "God, I had an accident", and sometimes you have to clean them up. It's the day-to-day stuff that's the hard part. By the time they get around to dying, it's almost easy. It's not easy, and it's sad, but the things you have to do to them while they're living are much harder than watching them die.

The work takes a tremendous toll, but it's not long lasting. When a patient came back after a weekend pass, I had to screw up my courage to tell him that we needed a toxic screen. He had to pee in a bottle so we could make sure that he wasn't drug-abusing. This guy had maybe six weeks to live, so who cares about the drug use! But this is one of our policies that we do whether he has six weeks or six months to live. I had to ask him for his cigarettes and matches again, even though he had been out for a weekend and had not burned himself up. When he was here, though, he burned a hole in his bed clothes and in his mattress. The risk hadn't changed over the weekend. Still, it was hard to ask for his cigarettes again. It gave me an instant headache. He didn't make a scene, but he was sad. He said, "I'm so tired, and now I have to walk up here to get my cigarettes."

We strip people of their independence all the time. This man is medicated quite often for pain, which can disorient him. It's not that he's being extra careless. He has no control over this anymore. I can't allow him to burn himself up.

Grilled Cheese Sandwiches and Saying Good-Bye

I get sentimental. The other day, we were thinking of a patient who lived on grilled cheese sandwiches for months. We started cancelling some of his regular food trays. Making him several grilled cheese sandwiches each shift was part of our care plan. As we were recalling this, we couldn't think of his name. I went back through hospital records of three years to find it. Those of us who had been here a while had a field day looking at past nursing assignments saying, "Oh, yeah, I remember him. Remember what this one used to do?" Sometimes it was good, and sometimes it was bad.

For me, reviewing the records of some former patients was a good feeling because the unit was fairly new, and I tended to remember the good parts. We took care of one guy who was severely demented. He would get dressed at three o'clock in the morning and say, "I'm going for my dental appointment now." It was hard to keep him off that elevator. Sometimes we even had to get security to bring him back. Now that he's gone, we remember his adventures as being cute. It wasn't cute at the time when we were right in it.

I've been to one funeral and one wake since I've been here. That's another part of my trying to separate myself. If I'm on duty when the person dies, I say my goodbyes when I'm doing up the body. We also have memorial services here, which I don't attend. I feel that I did my best when they were alive, and now they're gone. We do have memories, though. We have a scrapbook that has fallen into disuse. We take pictures and write comments. There are a lot of things that are done around here that might be seen as morbid, but I think it helps us reach a feeling of closure. We talk about our deceased patients quite frequently.

We remember a little something about almost everybody that we've taken care of. Sometimes, it helps us treat other patients. The symptoms appear over and over. We'll say, "Remember what we did with Mr. So and So? This patient is acting like that, maybe we'll try that. Maybe that will work." This is how our basic knowledge and experience is built up. When I get sentimental, I say that this is their gift to us because their treatment and experience made us wiser.

I'm Careful So I'm Not Afraid: The Security of Gloves

I haven't gotten stuck with a dirty needle since I've been here, knock on wood, although I've been stuck in my nursing career. They weren't testing for AIDS at that point, and I got a pretty dirty stick from a guy who had open heart surgery. He had multiple transfusions of blood from God knows where, and I used to think about that. I went through a really bad period of thinking about that a lot.

I'm not afraid of catching anything from these guys. We have a lot of people with herpes here, and I'm careful with that. I'm careful so I'm not afraid. We'll talk to each other: "If you're going in there, use gloves. Don't think you're impervious. You're not Superman. You're not

Superwoman." Patients even take care of us. A lot of them will say, "Hey, why don't you put some gloves on."

I used to think that we were really special, and I don't really feel that anymore. When this unit started, it was all volunteers because there was so much AIDS phobia and homophobia. With the advent of universal precautions, if you're careful and you're not in the wrong place at the wrong time, you're not going to get AIDS. Years ago, we would have been the medical staff who worked with people with Hansen's disease (leprosy) or in TB sanitariums.

Coping with AIDS Work

I have to look at my work in eight-hour blocks because sometimes the day can be so hideous. Sometimes it's patient-related and sometimes staff-related. The stress is pretty high on the staff, and we really have to make an effort to let it go at the end of the day. An effort has to be made not to obsess on it. You have to find something else to do that is going to take your mind off what you were doing on the AIDS unit that day.

I try to manage one situation at a time. Some situations are much easier to let go of than others. Some of them I can rationalize away. A man was terribly angry at me because he didn't get his two fried eggs. Another man was terribly angry at me because his pain wasn't being managed well. I look at the first instance and say, "Toss off the fried eggs. We can do something about that." For the second problem, we may need to have a conference. Maybe we need to talk to him more. There are things to obsess on and things not to obsess on. I try to get a balance. Sometimes I'm successful.

I'm a natural worrier. I used to go to bed and lie there before I went to sleep, giving myself a report again. Sometimes, it made me feel good because I gave myself a report, and everything was taken care of. Other times, it didn't make me feel good because I'd say, "Geez, I forgot to do this. I forgot to do that. I should have gotten to this for this patient. I didn't call in that referral to another therapy."

Sometimes, I feel guilty about trying to let it all go. I tell myself that I should stay and do this paperwork. I should stay and work on this one more chart. I cheat myself when I do that. I tell the nurses that if you did your eight hours well, there's no reason why you shouldn't go home and do something else. I've sent nurses off the floor telling them, "You need to put on your coat and go outside for ten minutes, and you can scream in the park." Sometimes, I just need to get away from the situation. Sometimes I can cope with it and let it go, and other times, I obsess on it even though it doesn't help.

I can't vent very much at home about my work. My family only partially approves of the job. My husband and I have always been very supportive in our professions. My mother was absolutely horrified that I was doing this. She has since gotten better. My kids were kind of so-so.

I think women listen better than men. If I come home with a problem, I'd better get it stated in five minutes or less or the interest rate goes way way down and that glazed look comes across their eyes. If I have a specific staff problem, I ask my husband, who has been in management longer than I have. If it's a nursing problem, I keep it in here. At work, you can grab somebody and say, "I need to scream or I need to go outside and walk around."

I've taken mental health days. I always feel guilty about calling in because I can't say I'm burned out and can't

take another day of this. I have to call in sick. Actually, I'm
not calling in sick, I'm calling in smart. Maybe I wouldn't
be good that next day because I might be on the edge of
screaming at the staff or at a patient. If you had such a
hideous day that you don't think you can take another
minute, maybe taking a day off or calling in sick in conjunc-
tion with your day off is going to allow you to come back
renewed. However, if someone wants to transfer off the unit
because they're burned out, I never encourage them to stay.
By the time a person thinks of leaving, they probably ought
to go. We've had staff members who have become burned
out and left.

I don't do formal exit interviews, but I always want
to find out why someone is leaving. Are you feeling unsup-
ported? Is it something in this population that drove you
away? Is it something that we could have done better? Were
you trying to tell us something, and we weren't listening?
Some patients are very difficult to take care of. We try to
split them up among staff members. If you keep giving
difficult patients to the same nurse, the nurse is going to get
burned out.

The families of the nurses are also affected by this
work. If you get stuck by a dirty needle, you have to
practice safe sex. A lot of significant others have gotten
burned out by this. In the interview, I ask how their family
or significant other feels about their working here. If we
find somebody who has people at home with very strong
negative feelings, we advise against working in our unit
because the job itself is hard enough. You need to be able to
go home and say two or three things about your work.

Here, we have one place to go with problems — a
support group where that kind of thing is monitored. You're
there with your peers and a group facilitator who is a

psychiatric liaison nurse. I don't go to the support group because management can't go, for fear of inhibiting the staff. I can see the group leader one-on-one. In the group, though, the nurses validate each others' feelings sometimes or tell you that you have to pull back, if you have the wrong perspective. This is one of the things that helps us, but sometimes there is no help. I encourage people to go to the support group, but not everyone goes. If we get them in there, they see that they're not operating in a vacuum. Sometimes, you can feel very alone, especially if you have a special attachment to a patient. If the patient isn't doing well, you're not doing well. You really internalize it.

There's a way to continue to do this work. Be with your kids. Try to decompress on the ride home. Read something stupid. Look at something on TV. Go to a movie. Whatever. I read, look at TV, do needlepoint, and talk to my cat.

Knowing Thyself

Working with people with AIDS makes me happy that my family and I are healthy. That's one of the selfish things that I say every day. I've been married for almost thirty years. I would hate it if I were out there dating now. I worry about my kids, especially my son because he's twenty-five and is dating. My daughter has been in a monogamous relationship for four years.

I'm a stickler. My husband always said that his life would be hell on earth if I couldn't get out my love of fixing details at work. He's probably right. I don't put hospital corners on the bed at home, but nursing is one of the places where you need to dot all the i's and cross all the t's. I enjoy doing that. This is a perfect outlet for it here, which is maybe why I'm finding that I'm good at it.

I'm also a nag. I try not to talk to the staff as though they were my family and my kids. I tend to fall into that mode because I'm older than most of them. I started nursing when I was older, and I'm more relaxed with it. I feel gratified if the floor runs well, the staff is happy, and there's been no patient crisis. Not every day is smooth, but if it happens a couple of times a month, it's enough to keep me going.

Chapter Six

Dennis: Separating the Disease from the People

I wanted to be involved in something that I believed was important and necessary.

Dennis has worked as a social worker for two years, including the past year and a half working with people with AIDS. In the past year, he's worked with thirty AIDS patients in a long-term hospital. He is a twenty-eight-year-old, white, heterosexual man.

Sometimes, he feels like a square peg in a round hole. New in his profession, Dennis is creating a place for himself. When he began working in his current position, staff members didn't understand his role. They thought he'd be filling out forms to get services and funding, and he had to teach them that he had emotional, therapeutic, and clinical skills to help the patients.

Dennis doesn't fit in perfectly with a community group of social workers who also work with AIDS patients.

Most of the members are women. Of the few men, the majority are gay.

He tries to make his personal life more ordered because his professional life can be so chaotic. It helps give him the stability he needs. His fiancé is generally supportive of his work with people with AIDS, but she has also voiced her underlying anxieties.

When he is able to separate the people from the disease, Dennis feels good, warmed, and rewarded to support patients who are often struggling with intense, painful life experiences. At times, though, he is unable to separate the disease entity from the people it affects and feels exhausted and sad. That's when he minimizes his patient contact.

Making a Place for Myself

When I came to this hospital, staff members thought social workers were here to do Medicaid and Social Security applications — very concrete, forms-oriented work. I had emotional, therapeutic, and clinical skills to contribute. I needed to educate them and make a place for myself.

In other areas, I'm still searching for my place. Sometimes, I feel guilty for being heterosexual. Many gay men and lesbians have become involved in AIDS care, and occasionally, someone assumes that I'm gay. I feel like I'm almost betraying them when I tell them I'm not. My sexual preference has made an impact on my work, although I don't feel that I'm treated differently. Maybe it's because I don't feel part of the group. In college, I had many gay and lesbian friends. I've been through a process of trying to become sensitive to the issues in their lives. In a professional setting, I've run into situations where I don't know what the sensitive and right thing is to do. It's still foreign to me.

I meet once a month with a group of social workers who work with AIDS patients. They're predominantly women. Of the men who are there, three or four out of five are gay. We talk about feelings and educate each other about resources and research. It crosses boundaries, and I don't always know how to deal with the situation. I move between different worlds at different times.

I like my work, and it's important to me. As much as that makes me feel good, I don't want to become pigeon-holed as an AIDS worker. It's early in my career, and I have a lot of working years ahead of me. I'm still hesitant to feel like I'm closing doors and choices.

Challenges and Learning

I chose to work with people with AIDS. I didn't want to work with adolescents any more and looked for an area with adults. AIDS care fell very much into that.

AIDS is a very different disease from other diseases treated in hospitals. As a terminal illness, there are emotional and family issues involved. It's also an illness that still has a great deal of perceived social consequences for the person with AIDS, the family, partners, friends, children, and spouses. We struggle with how to provide for the great range of client needs within the limitations of working under a medical model.

We're dealing with long-term IV drug users. We're dealing with people who have never developed adequate coping mechanisms for crises in their lives. They come from families with poor communication skills. Many have been abused and/or abuse others. Even the gay men may not have received a lot of family acceptance and support before becoming sick. Their sexuality and partners may have been denied family approval even though there may have been family contact. There's always this extra set of needs.

We do pretty well with dealing with these needs, but we haven't reached the point where we do it right. We provide high quality care and treat our patients as humans, which says a lot for us as a program and as people. There's still more to do, though. We need to explode our professional boundaries and learn to work with others.

My work with people with AIDS is challenging, rewarding, sad, and thought-provoking. Dealing with the daily emotional reactions of clients, staff, and myself is the most challenging aspect. There's an enormous amount of information, and it's continually changing. Every Monday, we have an hour research presentation about AIDS. Although I don't have a poor science background, some of this stuff is way over my head. I'm challenged by the amount of information that I don't know and how much I'm constantly having to learn.

I have to learn about the hospital. I have to learn about the Department of Corrections. I have to learn how to interact as liaison between the AIDS program and all the other systems. I have to learn about the state bureaucracy, and I need to learn about the disease. I need to learn about microbiology, tuberculosis, and pneumonia. I need to learn about what Medicaid defines as acute versus chronic levels of care. To complicate matters, some of this is always changing. That's really challenging!

There's so much involved in providing care to this group. Most of my previous work was with families and children. I need different skills as a social worker to work with this population. Working with issues of death and dying is professionally and personally challenging. It raises a lot of emotions for me. Dealing with my emotional reactions without them interfering with client relationships is a challenge.

Occasionally, I have fears about working in this environment — but not about contracting HIV. I'm waiting for my PPD (test for tuberculosis conversion) to be positive. During my second week here, I suddenly realized that I could catch something. As a social worker, I don't deal with needles or have any of the high-risk exposures to body fluids. That's the least of my worries. There are all these other illnesses floating around that I need to think about. My first patient was on respiratory precautions. I had to wear a mask to go in to talk to him. I had never done that. I have my moments when I'm apprehensive about medical things, mostly regarding things I know nothing about.

We had a small outbreak of MRS (methicillin-resistant staphylococcic infection). We all had to get cultured. Realistically, there's very little that I can catch here that's going to harm me in any long-term way. But when new things crop up, I'm a little apprehensive until I learn more about it.

Emotional Exhaustion and Endings

My relationships with clients generally begin by focusing on concrete issues, such as discharge planning, benefits, and entitlement programs. Throughout their hospital stay, I have the most intense contact around specific events or issues, like coordinating family visits, making arrangements around discharge plans, and mediating conflicts between patients and families.

When patients are here for a longer period of time, there may be a period in which there are no concrete issues that need to be addressed. I'll stop by to say hello and develop ongoing relationships. I'll continue to make sure that they're not having trouble with their insurance company, need arrangements at home, or want an AIDS buddy. The contacts become a little more casual and therapeutic. I can do some more emotional-based work with them. Since my office is on the floor with the patients, I know everybody and see them as they're walking around.

Some days, I see the people, and some days, I only see the disease. On the days that I see people as people, I have warm emotional reactions to working with courageous or frightened people who are struggling to face painful and intense experiences. It feels good to be a supportive part of that, especially when it's with clients who are improving. On the days that I see the disease, I feel very tired and am more hesitant to spend time with patients. On those days, I feel sad and exhausted and tend to put off contact with patients.

When I feel less personally supported in my life, I have less energy for patients and have fewer defenses against the sadness, dying, and the disease. My contact with patients isn't something that often gives me strength in and of itself. I get strength because I feel good about the work I'm doing. When I'm sad, I don't turn to our patients to make me feel better.

Sometimes, the work becomes exhausting. Several patients may die one right after another, two or three people in a week. At times, I work exceptionally hard with difficult discharges, making arrangements for the patients to go to hospice or get services at home. When I have those endings, especially many at once, I feel exhausted. I feel drained with too much closure and don't have a lot of energy to put into new contacts.

I don't necessarily get closure when a person dies or is discharged. With some of our discharged clients, we usually know whether we'll see them again. If my relationship with clients has been mostly professional, I feel that my work has been wrapped up at their death or discharge. That becomes a comfortable closing. If there has been more emotional contact or I feel my professional work hasn't been completed because of running out of time, for example, it's very unsatisfying.

When patients die, there's less closure, and I feel a greater loss. A gentleman came here last October and stayed for six months. When he was first admitted, he was very communicative. His legs were extremely weak, and he couldn't walk much. He got around in a wheelchair and became involved with people. A number of times, he went down to chapel and sang services with the chaplain. By the time he left, he was very debilitated and wasted, could barely talk, and was on a morphine drip.

When I was completing the social service referral form for his transfer to hospice, I became aware of how important it was to me that the hospice staff know what a beautiful singer he was. That wasn't a very professional thing for me to put on the form, but how else would they know the person behind the person? I ended up not including it. He was transferred and died a week later.

Making a Difference — Feeling Effective

A patient, who had been in the hospital for three or four months, had been in prison for a number of years before that. He hadn't been in touch with his mother for ten years. She spoke no English, lived somewhere in the Bronx, and was in a wheelchair since her stroke. I managed to track her down and write a letter in Spanish, which took a great deal of time. She received the letter and called her son. I felt very good and effective about that. I put in a lot of time and energy, and it worked. It was a very positive interaction for mother and son.

I feel effective when my being here makes a difference. I connected with a woman whose daughter was our patient for months. The mother was involved in the daughter's care and was having a difficult time dealing with the fact that her daughter was going to die. She was a very spiritual woman who put a lot of faith in her prayers that her daughter would have one more recovery and be able to come home. It became clear that it wasn't going to happen. I spent time with the mother over the course of the daughter's last week of life. I didn't do anything concrete for her mother, but I felt that what I was doing was very important.

When the mother ran out of the room because it became too painful for her, I was there. When she needed to talk, I was there. I gave her a place to review her life with her daughter and begin to have some perspective on her daughter's dying. She began to look toward the future without her daughter. The mother was taking care of her daughter's child and that was part of going on with life. There were a lot of life and death transitional issues for her. I was doing something for her that nobody else was.

Anger + Frustration = Ineffectiveness

A patient who was at a very late stage in his disease wanted to believe that he was going to get better again. I felt that he wanted me to say, "Everything's going to be okay. You're getting better." There's a fine line between fueling fantasies and stopping hope. I felt that it was important to say, "You might get better in the short term, but you still have an illness that isn't going to go away." It really wasn't what he wanted to hear. Even though I felt honest about what I was doing, I felt that I wasn't being effective. I wasn't providing something positive to him, which is the same thing as not being effective.

Another patient, who had been here for more than a year, just went home to her daughter's house. Although that's a great success because we never thought it was going to happen, it's a very disorganized, chaotic family — the patient, her daughter, the daughter's two children, and the daughter's partner. I met with them several times over the past six months, but we're not a family service agency. We have no mechanism to provide ongoing family therapy and no hook to make the family participate. We can't say, "You can't see your mother unless you talk to me first every time you come in." It's not part of our mission. The family isn't any more organized now than they were when I started working with them. What I did wasn't bad, but I certainly didn't feel effective.

I also felt very frustrated and angry. As much as I hate to say this, I also felt a little self-righteous. I had seen what was wrong, gave them my time, skills, and access to some tools, yet I couldn't get them involved in that sort of relationship with me. They never wanted to utilize me or the rest of the staff to benefit themselves. There were times I felt like twisting their arms by saying, "You can't take your mother out on a pass until you start doing this for her." To force them into a contract would have been punitive.

The majority of our patients are IV drug users or have a history of substance abuse. Typically, they are part of very disorganized families with multiple problems, needs, and issues. Sometimes, I feel mad at them because of the pain they've inflicted on other people. This hits me especially hard when they've used their illness to run the family or create an environment where their children's emotional needs are not recognized or fulfilled.

One of our patients had gone on a drinking binge, aspirated, and got pneumonia. He was admitted here but left the hospital against medical advice a week before his treatment was finished. Three weeks later, he did the same thing. He was readmitted for about a month of antibiotic treatment and rehab but left four days before the end of the treatment. We saw him a third time and heard he was later admitted to two other hospitals for the same thing. We each wanted to say, "If you don't stop this, you're going to die." It takes a lot of anger for me to reach that point. I wouldn't say it lightly.

I'm also angry when our patients are denied access to resources or are snubbed by their family, friends, or correctional institutions. They have AIDS and may be poor, uneducated, drug addicts, without a work history — all things people look down on. When they're here, I look past a lot of that and get a chance to see people as human beings. Everyone here gets up in the morning, brushes their teeth, and wants little things in life, whether it's having a cigarette or walking to the kitchen by themselves to get a cup of coffee. They're just like anybody else, but there are institutions, agencies, or people who are unable or unwilling to see that aspect of them.

Painful Professional Experiences Trigger Personal Responses

I still have painful experiences at work that trigger personal responses. An older patient reminded me of the way my father looked not long before he died. It stirred up a lot of feelings over a great and painful loss, including aspects that I buried or tried to shield myself from. It caused me to let a little more of that pain into my life. I also connected to this patient in a different way and felt a little sadder about him.

It's also painful for me to have to be bluntly direct with people to help them deal with difficult situations. When patients have a terminal illness, family members often don't want to deal with it. I don't want to give them an excuse for putting off emotional issues that they need to work out with the patients. When patients want to talk about where and how they wish to be buried, family members often say, "We'll have lots of time to deal with this." There may be a lot of time, but they can't count on it. They need to face this now. I find that very difficult.

The doctor has to tell so many people painful things. I'm shielded from a lot of that because I'm not the one who gives medical advice. I'm not the first contact, but I am a contact. Even after a patient has been told, "You're at the end of your illness now," often they will say to me, "The doctor says I'm at the end of my illness, but I don't think so." I tell them, "Maybe you're right, but maybe you ought to think about what she said." They look at me thinking, "Uh-oh, if he's saying this...." That's very hard. I'm inflicting sadness, and it's a painful thing for me to do.

Coping is a Balancing Act

I'm in a unique position here. Although the schedule fluctuates, my administrative duties and patient responsibilities are each supposed to account for half of my time. The administrative stuff offers me a much greater buffer, a distraction from patient issues. It probably saves me from being continually overwhelmed. I'm responsible for a fairly well-defined piece of care, unlike the nurses, doctors, and physician assistants — people who deal with patient care all the time. They tell the patients about their physical condition, help them get dressed, take baths, lift them. I couldn't do that. I don't have what it takes emotionally to provide that physical care.

At first, I tried to split my work and home life. When I was at work, I worked, and when I was at home, I didn't do work. It didn't work! Working with people with AIDS stirs up emotions that I take home in different ways. I also bring emotions from home to work. I have to learn how to filter the emotions so that they don't overwhelm the other part of my life. I don't always do it effectively.

My fiancé has some concern about my working with people with AIDS. When I started, she joked that I couldn't go around kissing my patients. I think that's reflective of her underlying anxieties. Generally, she's supportive. She respects my work and recognizes that it's important. That makes coping with this work a little easier.

Initially, I was really excited about my new job and would tell people about it. They'd say, "What you do is so hard, how can you work with AIDS patients?" Or they'd ask me something about AIDS. My widowed aunt, in her mid-to-late sixties, asked me whether she and her boyfriend needed to use condoms. I felt very awkward and uncomfortable. When people are looking for basic AIDS education, I tell them that they ought to talk to someone who can give them attention and answer all their questions. I don't want to do that with friends or acquaintances. I no longer want to talk about my work when I'm not at the hospital. I had to learn where the limits are, how to set them, and how to own my feelings.

When I go home, I usually try to do something of low emotional content that lets me air out a little bit — read the paper, watch the news or the game. From the time I leave on Friday until I return to work on Monday, I have twenty thousand things that I have to get done, but I try to make room to play.

I put a lot more effort into making sure my world outside of work is unchaotic. I need some order in my life. Every week, I try to set one goal for home, and I have done a fairly good job keeping to that. I wanted to try some cooking, and I did. I like to visit with people, so I do. I have to do my laundry. Those little things provide me with some stability. That's probably the key to it. I have to work at keeping a balance in my life between my AIDS work and personal arenas.

Chapter Seven

Steve: Identifying with the Patients

I have a whole realm of feelings. There's lots of happiness, lots of fun, and lots of sadness. There's some anger and feelings of identity. It could very easily be me!

Steve is a thirty-eight-year-old, white, homosexual man. A physical therapist with fourteen-and-a-half years of experience, he has worked with people with AIDS for five of those years. This past year, he treated ten patients with AIDS in an acute private hospital.

Being openly gay, Steve feels that he can better understand many of the issues that his patients face. He belongs to a gay runner's group and marches in the Gay Pride parade. He's a man who's comfortable with himself.

Unlike some of the other health professionals I spoke with, Steve doesn't primarily work with people who have low education, poor finances, a drug history, or a criminal record. His identification with the white, upper class, middle-aged, gay male patients he treats is the most painful for him. It causes him to prematurely face issues of his own mortality and that of his friends. "There but for the grace of God go I."

As a physical therapist, he works to limit disability and restore physical function. Most conditions and diseases have a linear progression, but AIDS has an unpredictable roller coaster that's difficult for Steve to deal with. It's a case of struggling forward and sliding backwards. Although Steve is saddened by caring for people along the continuum of life to death, he finds his work very validating as a caregiver and as a human being.

A Whole Realm of Feelings

Working with patients with AIDS is professionally challenging and emotionally draining. It also makes me feel good being able to help people who really need help. It's incredibly gratifying when I can get someone back to a functional level so that he or she can go home from the hospital.

Even though I'm working with a group of people whose outlook is not great, I look at the small picture rather than the larger picture. The large picture is rather gloomy because I see these people coming back to the hospital, each time being a little worse. The small picture is helping them get over the present crisis, in the short-term, so that they're able to get back to living their lives on the outside. There's really a lot of satisfaction in helping that process along and getting them home.

A little bit of fear stays in the back of my mind so that I'm cautious and prevent infection. If I'm treating a patient with no open wounds or incontinence, I don't wear gloves or gowns, and I touch the patients. I get real close to them. I talk to them. If I'm working around open wounds or doing exercises with someone on bedrest with copious diarrhea, I wear gloves. If I help change a patient who has had an accident while I'm in the room, I'll put a gown over my clothes just to protect them, since this involves turning the patient and coming into contact with dirty sheets. If I employ universal precautions with every patient like I'm supposed to do, I cover all my bases and don't really have to worry about it.

This work challenges all aspects of my personality. Professionally, I utilize all the skills I have as a physical therapist to do the best job that I can for patients. I know full well that most of the improvements I make will be short-term. It's also a challenge to me personally. Most of these individuals are in my age group, the greatest percentage of them share my same sexual orientation, and some of them are my friends. I feel good lending professional expertise and emotional support to make their lives easier.

I heard my name called as I walked through the chemotherapy clinic the other day. A patient came over and gave me a big hug and a big kiss right in the middle of the chemo clinic. I had treated him in private practice, and now he was at the hospital for treatment of lymphoma. He really needed someone to sit and talk with him. Instead of continuing upstairs, I sat and talked with him for a half hour. Being able to provide that kind of support, within the context of being a professional and a caring individual, made me feel good about what I'm doing. The down side is the sadness that goes with that. A lot of people I really care about have lost their lives, and several more are on their way, including those I don't yet know. My experience covers the whole continuum of emotions.

I've worked in this field long enough to have learned how to protect myself from getting emotionally involved with patients. It's too devastating to do that on a regular basis. I vividly remember a couple of patients who I saw early in their disease progression. Following them over the long-term and seeing them deteriorate was rather painful.

We see a skewed population of AIDS patients at this hospital. They tend to be mostly white, upper class, middle-aged, gay men — a group that I identify with quite significantly. This is the most painful part of the experience for me. Whenever I see one of these people, it's like seeing one of my peers, one of my friends, or even myself — having to face death and dying issues in the prime of life. That's a very tough thing to spend a lot of time dwelling on.

Perspectives on Making a Difference

One of the first patients with AIDS that I worked with was a young man who had primary lymphoma. His outlook wasn't good. It was questionable whether he would be able to go home with his family, lover, and lover's parents taking care of him. Through my work with him, he was able to go home, ambulating with a cane. Everyone was so happy that this gentleman was going to be able to die in his own home with his family nearby. I felt great helping him get to that point!

At a private practice where I also work, I treated an HIV-infected patient who had musculoskeletal problems unrelated to his HIV. I was able to help solve some of his problems, making him more comfortable and able to return to work. He gave me positive feedback on the changes that occurred as a result of our interaction. That was pretty significant!

There was one young man who was married and had children. I can't remember how he became infected, but I started working with him when he had a severe bout of PCP (pneumocystis carinii pneumonia). He ended up in the intensive care unit on a ventilator, which he was fighting all the way. They had to use a drug to paralyze him. In some people, it has a slow weaning effect, and he had severe muscle weakness for a long time afterwards. In addition, he had painful herpes lesions rectally. Progressing him from being bedbound on a ventilator to getting out of bed and sitting in a chair to walking with a walker was a very effective experience. He went to rehab before going home. Taking someone who was incapacitated with so many problems and getting him to a fairly significant functional level, one step closer to going home, was fantastic!

I treated a patient with significant KS (Kaposi's sarcoma) on both legs and cellulitis on one leg. We accomplished the goal of getting him ambulatory so that he could go home with visiting nurse services. A week later, he was back in the hospital because he had developed significant weakness in the leg without cellulitis and could no longer walk with his walker. He had developed vacuolar myelopathy, bowel and bladder incontinence, and paraplegia around the waist level. Every day I encouraged him to focus on whatever he had left, but every day I could see that he had less and less. While I was encouraging him to be positive and focus on what he had, all I could really see was how much he was losing. He ended up getting PCP and died here in the hospital. That was one of those incidences where I didn't feel like I was really doing much for him. On the upside, I'd like to think that our daily interactions were okay for him and encouraged him to be positive as long as he could.

As a physical therapist, one of the problems I have working with AIDS patients is that I tend to look at linear progress. I make an intervention, and if I'm good at what I do, the person benefits and gets better. That doesn't always work with AIDS patients. In the short run, they may get better from the intervention and go home, but they come back in worse condition. Two steps forward and three steps backward. I have to work at letting go of that.

Surrounded by Illness — Lessons, Changes, and Burnout

I've learned that I can't do too much about the past and really have no control over the future, so there's no point worrying about either one. What is important is happening right now, today, a philosophy that comes out of facing death and dying. Having a number of friends who have died and knowing the number of people who have HIV — and knowing that I could very well be in that same position — has brought this home for me. This is probably the biggest thing that I've learned and tried to change in my life.

My sexual preference has made me more passionate about my work. One of the problems I see is that even though the AIDS care is very good at this hospital, most of it is done by straight people. I've heard numerous stories of some of the caregivers' negative remarks about homosexual lifestyles and IV drug use. Although the comments are made behind closed doors and not in front of the patients, some of the emotions behind them must come through. My identity with the gay subgroup has made me a little more enthusiastic about wanting to get involved. It also provides the individuals with some level of interaction that they don't usually get on a regular basis. I can appreciate what it's like to leave a mother or some parts of the gay life behind and am able to converse on that level while treating the patients.

I've noticed changes in my work as I gain experience and get older, but unfortunately, they're not very positive. I'm getting tired being a cheerleader for the population. I'm also getting tired of trying to get people to do things that they don't want to do, such as changing cardiovascular risk factors. I definitely feel like I'm burned out.

I still have some desire to work exclusively with the AIDS population, to work in a hospice for AIDS patients and really get to know and interact with these people on a much deeper level than I get to do here. I don't understand it. On one hand, I'm talking about being burned out in health care, but on the other hand, I'm talking about putting myself in a situation where burnout is even a higher risk. Working through hospice, you don't necessarily have to be a cheerleader. It's a different process. You're preparing someone to accept the end of this stage of their life. You're not goading them to make significant changes in their lives so that they can prevent their dying. I think that it's an experience that I would like to have.

I feel as burned out as I did six months ago when I started worrying about being burned out. Doing many different things during the day relieves some of the pressure. I'm able to remove myself from the situation for a short period of time — waste fifteen minutes, go for a walk, head to the cafeteria, look at the sports page for fifteen minutes — and regroup before I return to what I was doing. I also talk to a number of people on the staff on a fairly regular basis.

I laugh a lot. I keep myself active socially. I exercise. I meditate. I bake bread. I have lots of coping mechanisms. I'm also in a position here at work where I do lots of different things during the day so I no longer spend my whole day treating patients. That's a big help!

Judgment, Education, and Caring

We're fighting the virus, not a group of people or a lifestyle. Gay men, prostitutes, IV drug abusers, and other people did not ask for this disease any more than any other supposedly innocent victims asked for it. A lot of that has to do with people's homophobia and their general feelings about certain lifestyles. It makes some people feel safer and more comfortable to point fingers.

I haven't heard of any nursing or professional staff member here who has refused to treat people with AIDS, but some maintenance workers and housekeeping people were reluctant to go in and clean the rooms after the patients had been there. The hospital really does a very good job educating its staff. They offer four or five AIDS Grand Rounds every year and several department inservices to educate individuals. The only way to stop people's fears is to educate them so that they feel like they have some knowledge and control over the situations that they're putting themselves in.

Health professionals who have a lot of negative feelings about homosexuality or people who use drugs need to get over it or find someone else to treat the patients. These patients are suffering so many other losses that they don't need to put up with uncaring or hostile caregivers. Health care providers need to educate themselves about accepting people for who they are and not being judgmental about other people's lifestyles. It certainly shouldn't affect their work.

I'm on a small public relations gambit. I'm not involved with ACT UP! I do march in the Gay Pride parade. I run with a gay group in town. I live my own life the way I want. I don't get into big rallies. I don't really worry about what people think of me. Maybe this is to my detriment. I probably don't protect myself enough. If I can educate people by having them meet me and see how comfortable I am living the life that I live with the friends that I have, I'll be achieving what I need to do at a personal level.

Chapter Eight

Ann: Painfully Sad Watching Them Fade

I still have a problem with how young most of them are. I'd be a liar if I said I don't feel sad, because sometimes I just do.

Fifty-four-year-old Ann is a white, heterosexual woman, with thirty years of nursing experience. During the past seven years, she has worked with AIDS patients, caring for more than one hundred in the past year in a long-term state hospital.

Instead of working as a staff nurse assigned to one unit, Ann travels throughout the hospital, coordinating patients' care to ready them for discharge. She arranges services, equipment, and referrals for the patients, as well as taking care of special needs to improve the patients' quality of life.

As much as she continues to be excited about her accomplishments, she often feels little joy in her work. The good news is that she loves being autonomous as she goes around the hospital. The downside of that solitary work is that she also feels lonesome, not connected to colleagues.

The more Ann struggles to get services for the clients, the more she gets frustrated. Everything becomes a major project — nothing comes easily. During our discussion, I sensed how tired she was, sagging under the weight of the world she carried on her shoulders. She told me that although she feels burned out, she still likes her work. When she began to work with people with AIDS, she was determined to treat them like all other patients. She got angry at hospital staff members who didn't even want to go into their rooms. She would make a difference.

Now that she's so tired, she has nowhere to go with it. Her family and friends don't want to hear about her work. She has no husband or companion to talk with. She can't find anything relaxing to do and blames herself that she hasn't taken care of her own needs.

Sadness pervades Ann's work, and she is particularly affected by the typically young age of her clients.

"It's Never Too Late to Make a New Friend" — Sadness, Pain, and Loss

Working with AIDS patients is gratifying, but it's primarily sad. If I had to describe it in one word, I'd say "sad." Everyone is so young. A lot of them have so much hope, and I know where it's going to end. When I meet a new client, I know that they're going to be my client for just x amount of time. It's gotten better, though, because people are living longer. That's good, but there's still no cure. Most of the clients know that, too, once they accept it.

I try to be outwardly hopeful, but inside, I know that our time together is going to be limited. I try to focus on the quality of life that they have now rather than on their expectation that there may be a cure in a hurry and they will get better very soon. I have to help them deal the best way they can and emphasize what's going on now, what they need to do, and what can make them more comfortable.

I never felt uncomfortable with people with AIDS. I always felt that it was a population that needed special attention and special help. I didn't have a problem with their sexual orientation. That's just a fact of life.

Watching somebody fade is painful. They get a little weaker, a little thinner, and maybe a little demented. I see this handsome young guy with a great personality. Maybe the next time I see him in the clinic, he seems like an old man, and I know that he's going to fade out. There's nothing I can do, and it's sad. Everybody is doing everything they can do, but it's not enough. It's sad with any disease, and there are a lot of terrible diseases. It's just with AIDS, there are so many of them all at once, and they're so young.

We see a lot of TB, with and without AIDS, and I say, "Oh my God, TB is everywhere." These diseases just keep coming, and it's pretty sad. Within the same client, of course, that's what the disease is, one infection after another.

It's very difficult to deal with these clients if you haven't had your own personal losses. If you haven't dealt with death yourself, it's hard to help someone else die or help their family deal with it.

Sometimes I get my ability to deal with loss from the clients. I stopped into a client's room one day and said, "Do you remember me? Do you mind if I come in and sit down and talk with you for a minute?" That man must have weighed about eighty pounds. He looked terrible. He said to me, "It's never too late to make a new friend." I thought, Oh, to think that he could say that and mean it! Gee, I wonder if I would be so pleasant or think to say that to someone if I were in his place.

Feeling Frustrated, Burned Out, and Ineffective

I feel frustrated about bureaucratic-type things. It's not always easy to get a service for the clients. They don't get their insurance quickly or there's no housing available. Everything's a job, a chore, and it's never just one phone call. It's a lot of phone calls. I might get it all in place and find out that the person lost his home. The whole thing can fall through. Sometimes, it's the clients who don't follow through on the one thing you gave them to do. That's really frustrating.

At first, a lot of hospital workers didn't want to deal with these patients. That made me angry, and I was all the more determined that I was going to deal with them and that they were going to be treated the same way as everyone else. It seemed like a disease that could be prevented if enough was done.

I'm feeling really burned out right now. I still like my work. There's nothing different that I want to do, but I need to do something for myself. I need to do something relaxing. I have to sit down and think about it. It's my own fault that I haven't done anything yet.

I don't feel very effective when someone won't speak to me, which happens occasionally. I try to understand where it's coming from and deal with it. If someone screams at me, it hurts and hits me in the face, especially if they say something nasty or their language is not what I'd like it to be. I realize that they're angry, upset that they're going to die, or having mental status changes. I've had the same thing happen with people I was trying to help who were alcoholics or drug users without AIDS. If they're not ready to accept my help and don't want to hear what I have to say, they tell me in no uncertain terms. I just walk away and leave it. Maybe they'll be ready another time.

I have plenty of family and friends, but no one wants to hear about AIDS or my work. Sometimes, we'll start talking, and I can tell people are thinking, "Oh no." They don't want to hear about it, so I just don't talk about it. It's very scary to them. Anyone can get it, and mostly young people get it. People just don't want to deal with that.

If anybody will listen, if I can corner somebody, I sometimes vent here at work. There is a support group for the staff nurses on the floor. Because I work all over the hospital, it probably wouldn't be geared to me, and I feel funny because I'm not part of that group and wouldn't belong. Typically, there's a bond between staff members on a floor because they're all doing the same things with the same patients every day. I go all around the hospital. I love the autonomy in my position, but it can be lonesome. If you're going to have that autonomy, loneliness is the price you pay.

"People Nobody Wants" — Choices, Challenges, and Excitement

The term "innocent victim" is ridiculous. It implies that if you got HIV through a blood transfusion, you're an innocent victim, but if you had a sexual encounter, you're not. That just puts up a wall. We're still hearing people say, "I don't think they should take all the money away from cancer research to save these people."

People are judgmental. They think about "this homosexual or this drug addict." If the person is a hemophiliac or someone who got infected through a transfusion, people just say, "Oh." It's sad no matter what.

I thought AIDS was going to be a big public health issue, and I thought it was very important. I felt that I could make a contribution and that it was needed. I don't exclusively deal with clients with AIDS, though it seems to be most of my clients. Before I was dealing with AIDS, I was still dealing with people with mental health problems and prisoners who were sick. I guess I felt good about that, too, because people don't want to deal with prisoners, and certainly, they don't want to deal with people who are mentally ill. They get treated worse than people with AIDS.

It seems to be a case of working with people nobody else wants. I knew what I was getting into. I had worked in the suburbs with middle-class people, and I gravitated toward the least desirable of people, if you could say there is such a category. To survive here, you have to know that and be able to deal with it. They're usually not too easy to deal with. Sometimes, I do something to someone, and they yell at me. Inside I know that I did the right thing, and it'll work out. Some people are not capable of saying thank you, but I do it for the good of society as a whole. Maybe they won't give this disease to somebody else.

So many people have jobs that are just "jobs," and they hate them. I feel lucky that I really haven't been in that position. I'm lucky that I have the opportunity to do this work. People ask, "How can you work with prisoners or mental health patients?" I say, "I like them." They're common folk. Some people are physically afraid to work with these populations. The needs of these clients are greater and more obvious. They're more of a challenge. A lot of these people don't have insurance, homes, significant others, all kinds of things. That's part of the challenge, being able to be creative. It's not just a job to me.

I get challenged by education. It's a big thing when I know somebody has listened to the education I gave them and is complying, like protecting themselves or their partner or doing what they're supposed to do. Most clients don't thank you. Because I'm not looking for them to thank me, I don't look for my satisfaction there. I like a challenge and am very determined.

It's hard to know if I am effective in educating people on a one-to-one basis because sometimes they "yes" me to death. But when I'm talking to a group, I can usually tell if I'm effective. Many people still believe that AIDS is restricted to one or two groups of people. Some middle-class organizations think that it's a gay disease or it's "those old drug addicts" who are going to give it to everybody else. They have a lot of preconceived ideas, and it's pretty hard to change their minds. When I win over a few of those die-hards, I feel pretty good.

It's really satisfying because there are so many needs. I get all excited when there are a lot of things that need to be done, and I can figure out a creative way to deliver that. It makes me feel good. The more of those needs I can fill for the clients, the more gratification I get. I usually can accomplish something for the clients — services, equipment, or referrals they need. That keeps me going. When I get a whole package of services together for someone or make a plan of theirs happen, I feel really satisfied. If I'm able to help somebody do something special for a child or partner before they die, I get a lot of return for that.

I try not to get too emotionally involved, at least that's been my rule. But I do become friends with them and get to know their families, girlfriends, husbands, or wives. So there is a connection. Sometimes, I identify with parents who are so devastated. I can just imagine what a parent is going through. A loss is a loss, but to lose a child...

I remember this woman who was dying. She had a little girl whom she hadn't been able to spend much time with. I went in one day and asked her how she was doing. She looked like she really wasn't doing well at all and said, "My little girl, I wanted to make her a Cinderella." I knew right away that she wanted to buy her a party dress and dress her all up. She was feeling really bad that she hadn't. It was too late, and it didn't happen. The next time there was a woman here and a child involved, I made sure that things like that happened. The woman didn't even have to say it. She didn't even think of it. Things like that are certainly gratifying and can make up for all the ones who scream "Get out of here."

Living with a Chronic Disease

I don't feel particularly scared or anxious, but I don't draw blood or give shots. If I did those things, I might feel a little anxious, but if you use good technique and do what you're supposed to do, there shouldn't be any problem. I certainly don't have any problem with touching or talking to a person.

It's easier for us now because people live longer. We used to get them in, and they'd get pneumonia and die. That doesn't happen anymore. There are people here who were diagnosed five and seven years ago. I told this gentleman yesterday that it's becoming more like a chronic disease. A person can live with that rather than knowing that this diagnosis means they're going to be dead within a month or two. You can live with the idea of a chronic disease because it means you can live.

They have hospice now, and I think they thought hospice was going to be full all the time because it's such a great concept. But it's very hard to be so young and have so much hope and say, "Enough, I don't want anything." It's difficult to do even if you're older, but when you're young, you think you're immortal. I see people practically taking their last breath saying, "Do everything. Try anything." Sometimes I can understand the fight, and sometimes I think the quality of their life is so miserable, and they're in such pain that I would understand if they gave up the fight.

I don't secretly hope that they give up the fight and die. Our doctors here are very good about pain control. They keep them really comfortable. If you can keep somebody comfortable and serene, that's the way it should be. If they're comfortable, they're not going to wish that they were dead.

The stigma, though, is terrible. Most families are so afraid that somebody is going to find out. What will the neighbors say? Most of them really don't have the courage to let it be known, so they don't get the amount of support they need. It's very difficult for them. I had a client, just the other day, who's known for a year or two that he was HIV-positive. He came to the clinic for some reason but never told the doctor here that he was positive. I asked him, "Why didn't you ever tell?" He said, "When I had the test, they said you don't have to tell anybody." I said, "Yeah, but if you had told the doctor, maybe he would have put you on AZT earlier." It's a big secret. His main concern was "How will I fill the prescription? They'll know," rather than "Gee, I might die."

Being afraid to be found out is a big issue because it affects whether they go for benefits or housing. They don't have access to many things because they're afraid to let anybody know. They're really taking a chance when they do let people know because people judge them right away.

Feeling Special — Advice for Other Health Professionals

I think that a lot of people are fascinated by this epidemic, what caused it, where it's going, how it gets there, and how it will end. I'm on the inside, exposed to all the new treatments and medicines as they come along. I've met different people from different backgrounds who have the disease, and I see how it has impacted their families and lovers. There are a lot of new experiences, and I can't help but grow and learn from it — and hopefully deal better with the next ones that come along.

There's something special about everyone, even a hardened criminal. He's a person and has other people in his life. If he doesn't and has burned all his bridges, it's nice to see him make some connection with his caregivers. It's kind of special, but you have to be very careful not to get too emotionally connected. You have to be able to keep it on a professional level or you couldn't do it for more than six months or a year. I've seen people last that long and not be able to continue doing it.

In my head, I know right up front that the clients will eventually die, and I think I deal with it better because I know that. As a provider, I don't think that you should get emotionally involved. I don't think it's healthy. I do feel sad and think of the significant other or children who are left behind.

I try to focus on something that I was able to accomplish while they were alive, like the time I helped a woman arrange something special to give her child a special memory. I felt sad when she died, but I remembered that special time that we were able to give that child. That helps me deal with it. I feel good that I'm able to help someone. Our clients are really needy.

I feel that maybe I have to take a break more often or maybe I have to do something for myself. I know I need to exercise or I need to do something constructive for myself, but I just don't do it a lot of times. I'm not a person who meditates or runs, but I need to learn to do something pleasurable — anything so I don't go home and think about my day.

I wouldn't do things outside of work with clients, and I wouldn't go to church services because it could just consume you. I've seen people leave after a short time, and I think that's why. You have to focus on what you can do to make things better for the clients and then be glad that you were able to do it. I guess that's the way I protect myself.

When someone dies, there's usually a small memorial service on the floor. The chaplain comes up, and they'll have a reading, sometimes a photograph of the person at some recreational event or something. I've only gone to one. I wouldn't go to a funeral or a wake. I would be going twice a week. I have to go to enough of them in my own life. See, that's where I have to draw the line. It would be too often and spill over into my personal life. It would be too devastating. I need to protect myself.

Chapter Nine

Laura: Coping with the Progressive Nature of AIDS

I have a morbid fascination with the disease.

Forty-six year old Laura is a heterosexual woman of color. A physical therapist for twenty-five years, she has worked in a pediatric neurology clinic with children with AIDS for five years, treating twenty such children in the last twelve months.

Passionate about pediatrics, Laura divides herself between clinical, research, and education roles. Over the years, she has developed stronger convictions about her patients' needs and is no longer reluctant to speak out. Working with children with AIDS is a significant part of her life, and yet, it can be taxing.

Laura is divorced, with no children. She appreciates the importance of support from her family and the man in her life with whom she enjoys a long-distance, committed relationship. When she's not working, she's able to release the strains of work by running, sailing, swimming, and other physical activities.

Initially, Laura chose to work with children with AIDS because they were segregated from other children, and no one else would treat them. She was angry at parents whose behavior led to the infection of their children. Now, she's learning to accept the human condition a little more, as well as the things she can't change.

Running and Valuing Life: Staying Balanced

I'm a runner. I can't wait for the summer with the heat, sailing, and swimming. I'm looking forward to that. I go to New York City to see the person that I adore. He's very supportive and knowledgeable about my work, so we can talk about it. Given the opportunity, I talk about it a lot. I've got a wonderful family whom I also adore. I feel very good about my life. Part of that carries over into what I do.

I don't really take credit for some of the good stuff that has happened to me, but I'll keep it. I can also appreciate that things haven't always been easy and wonderful for other people, nor does everyone have the strength to change the way things are going for them. I find it intolerable to live in a situation where I'm not comfortable or happy. We make our own life and our own choices. I've had some experiences where I've been miserable. Life is too short to be miserable. That's part of why I got divorced. I feel somewhat in control of my life and have responsibility for how it's going to be. If I don't like it, then I'll change it. If I'm happy with it, I'll try to keep prolonging those things because you never know when things are going to come and knock you for a loop.

I've always valued my life. I don't know that I've always valued other people's lives as much as I do now. It bothers me to see homeless people in New York. At one point, it didn't bother me if people on drugs died of an overdose. It was their own fault. I feel sad about that, but I no longer feel it's my responsibility to try to change everyone, to pick everyone up and dust them off.

Entering the World of Children and AIDS

Working with children with AIDS is no different from working with children with other disorders. I came into the field to provide training to therapists who were working with children with developmental disabilities. The children I first saw, before I knew their AIDS diagnoses, didn't look very different from other children with cerebral palsy or other neurological deficits. The thing that you have to cope with is the emotional sort of battle — knowing that it's a progressive disease that ends in death. The focus of my treatment, though, is being able to treat the neurological and developmental deficits in children. If part of the cause of that is HIV, it means going on a quest to find out how that disease manifests itself in the child that I'm seeing. The focus is not terribly different in the way that I treat any other child.

At one point, I made a conscious effort to work with children with AIDS. At a hospital in New York City, children with HIV infections weren't specifically earmarked for treatment in the acute care setting. It became a little bit more difficult for them to get their physical therapy services once they were diagnosed. Staff members were afraid to work with children with HIV and integrate them into the setting where there were other children. Initially, those children were segregated. I elected to treat them on an outpatient basis in the regular acute-care hospital. All the other children with developmental disabilities went to the developmental disabilities clinic. I was associated with both clinics, but initially, I was the only one who was treating these children because no one else would.

I knew what to do with children who were presenting with this clinical picture, but in 1985, I knew nothing about HIV infections in children. I knew how it was transmitted and how it impacted on adults, but I wondered what children were doing with AIDS. That was part of my research mind, starting on the quest to find out more about the disease.

Meeting with pediatricians and neonatologists, I said, "I understand we're seeing many children with HIV infections in the hospital. Why is it that we're not seeing them in rehab? They're more developmentally delayed. Why?"

"We don't know," they always answered. I suggested to all these pediatricians and neonatologists that they refer the children with HIV infections to me so that I could at least evaluate them and see if they needed treatment for their developmental deficits. In that way, we got them started into the system. After about two years of learning about the disease and fighting emotional battles with the people who were trying to discriminate, we were finally able to get the kids incorporated into the regular developmental disabilities clinic program.

People ask me how I can work with these poor little kids. Does it make me depressed? No, it doesn't depress me. I'm really more struck with the hope of how we can do something better. I find it a lot easier to treat children than adults with HIV. My feeling is more fatalistic with adults. It seems that they're dying faster or sooner than the children. Yet statistics show us that children naturally have a shorter latency period and their life expectancy is shorter. We have fewer choices about the medical intervention with children. I don't know what it is. I like kids better than I like adults.

As adults progress with the disease, they look worse. It's hard when the gauntness of the wasting syndrome and respiratory disorders take effect. It's easier for me to deal with the physiological progression of the disease in children than with the progressive motor and neurological dysfunction in adults. I can slow this down for a little bit in children, but I don't have the same feeling that I could stop this in adults.

Prior to the onset of the disease, adults presumably had normal motor function and now they demonstrate a loss. Children start off developmentally lower down and can build up. Whatever you do might be a gain. There's always something you can tap to make them better in some way.

Looking at the Child as a Child, Not a Disease: Feeling Effective

I can point most specifically to the first child with AIDS I ever treated on a regular basis. She was a little girl of eighteen months who was severely disabled. Diagnosed with AIDS at three months because she had PCP (pneumocystis carinii pneumonia), she had almost no righting reactions, was unable to sit independently, and had no mobility whatsoever. She had the most caring foster family I had ever seen. They were at their wits' end trying to figure out what they could do to help this child. I met with the foster mother and said, "What do you want me to help you with?" The mom said, "What can you help me do so that I can feed her? She used to eat more solid foods. She can't now and is losing weight. We're worried about her." These were the same concerns that any mother would have for her children whether they were handicapped or not.

The most exciting part was being able to work with the mother, father, sisters, cousins, uncles, and brothers who came in to see what the therapist was doing so that they could carry it out at home. This little girl, who fit into a relentlessly progressive category of encephalopathy, was able to make some changes. She developed some postural reactions and could be left alone on the floor, able to push herself up onto her arms, look at the other kids, and participate with the family. I showed them how to desensitize her mouth, how to put her on a feeding program, and introduce different foods so that she could eat better. She started to eat better, which made her grandmother much happier.

She died about ten or twelve months later, but during the time she was in treatment, she had a good solid seven or eight months of progress. I think that's one of the things that's exciting about physical therapy — helping families see that they can do something other than watch this child with a fatal disease die. They stop looking at the child as a disease and start looking at the child as a child.

Evaluations, Not Treatments: Frustrations and Painful Experiences

I'm in a different setting now and see children in a pediatric neurology clinic. I do evaluations, not treatments. I feel the most successful when I'm actually able to do treatments and see the outcomes of the treatments. In my current position of consultant and evaluator, I'm frustrated by seeing a child at one point in his or her development and knowing that I'm not going to be seeing them for treatment. When I see the child several months later with more debilitation, I think I could have made a difference. That's the most painful experience. I expect that's going to continue because I consult at two day care centers, and the numbers of children that we see in clinic are not necessarily going to be picked up for treatment.

It's different from knowing that I'm doing as much as I can do and that whatever negatives happen are due to the progression of the disease. I still have the feeling that I should be able to do something and have it make a difference. Each time I find out that it doesn't, it's painful. It's even more painful if I know that something could be done but that needed services didn't get to the child.

There was a child on the research protocol who had been having developmental assessments since he was three months old. At seven months old, the team said, "He's looking good. He's really improving. He's gaining in his developmental skills." They used a testing tool that I don't believe picks up quality of movement. The child is now twelve months old. I saw him yesterday with his mother. She had noticed that his legs are widely abducted (apart), he's starting to pull to standing, he's starting to walk, but he's markedly externally rotated (legs turned outward), with a very wide basis of support. She thinks he looks funny, and she doesn't want him stigmatized.

It's not a very good feeling to see a child of twelve months and know that he should have gotten treatment at seven months of age when we saw him. He wasn't doing well. He had a wide base of support then. He was delayed in his crawling. Even though the team, which was not made up of therapists, said he was doing very well in his development, I, as a therapist, did not speak out strongly enough and say that he wasn't doing well. He's still below where he should be in the quality of his movements, and that's going to have an impact, with his being more delayed over time. I didn't know enough to say that then.

We do see a wide base of support, and some children are slower than others in coming up into quadruped (on hands and knees) and onto their knees and making their transitions. Now, I say that treatment is important between the ages of six and ten months. Try to do something about righting reactions, postural reactions, and getting them up against gravity sooner than they would on their own. That's one thing that I feel the most guilty about so far.

I can say that I didn't know to take that strong a stand then, but I did take this stand yesterday. This child needs treatment now, and the mother needs to be taught what to do. I worked with the mother for about an hour. Then I met with her case worker and said, "Do you think that she had too much to do? Do you think she was too overwhelmed with the things that I was trying to tell her? How often is the child coming into the center so that I can make a point to see him?" The problems are still going to be there. He's not coming regularly into the center where I consult. The chances of my being able to follow through on what I'm saying are slim. He needs treatment now if he's going to look different, but I don't know if he's going to look different with treatment nor do I know the duration and frequency of treatment that's going to be important in order for him to change. Now, I'm willing to stick my neck out and say, "I think we can make a difference."

I haven't felt burnout so far, but I keep changing work locations. I was the sole person carrying all the children who had HIV infection where I worked in New York City, just me and the families. Of course, there were physicians who wrote referrals for physical therapy, but the day-to-day contact and the successes or failures of the child and family really fell on my shoulders. I didn't realize it at the time. Around the time that I was feeling like the voice in the wilderness, the developmental clinic became organized and formed a team to provide services.

In the centers where I now consult, I'm not the only person providing services on an ongoing basis. There are case managers, outreach workers, and family support systems for the families and the children. When I was the primary provider, I didn't realize how much of a responsibility it was. It's easier working with a team of people who are all dealing with the same issues. It was only after I left that setting that I realized how much I was doing and how much I was getting involved in their lives. I didn't want to do that anymore. I'm a physical therapist, not a counselor.

I think I would be burned out if I didn't feel I was effective. The most frustrating thing in the clinic for me now is when all they want me to do is take a look at a kid and write up an evaluation. They want a five minute evaluation on a motor problem when I can see that the child needs treatment to correct the problem. All they want is the evaluation. When I say, "This kid needs treatment. I'll do it," they tell me I can't. "Yes, I can. Yes I can. I can do this." That split between evaluation and treatment is a big source of frustration.

At least I know that the clinical research is helping and not going into an empty well. The information goes into a database which can be used to help other people. I know that there are going to be some kids five years from now that I'll think, "This would have worked with that kid," or "I was on the wrong track with that one." I sometimes feel frustrated because I don't have enough time to write down all the information that I feel should be put together. As long as I can keep putting this information together and sharing it with other people, more people are able to make more effective decisions. They don't have to go through the same sort of struggle that I did to come up with the answers. The other part of the frustration and pain is knowing there's only so much we're going to be able to do for a fatal disease. Part of me is beginning to realize that.

Fear, Anger, and Saving Lives

I've run the gamut of emotions. One of the first things I felt when I started working with children with AIDS was that physical therapy was going to save their lives. Of course, I realized that wasn't true. I just had the feeling that physical therapy would make a difference in stopping the progression of the disease. It doesn't.

I also felt the fear and the possibility of catching the disease because I didn't always wear gloves. I had questions, especially back in the early days. When I looked at a cut on my hands, I'd ask myself if I had that cut on my hand when I was treating this child. I used to do oral motor stimulation, but I wore gloves for that. Then there was the question about using latex gloves versus the other kinds of rubber gloves. Am I subjecting myself to the possibility of infection, not just from HIV but from other diseases and disorders kids have, like the skin diseases? I found that I'm susceptible to some of the bacteria and fungal infections they get. I get ringworm very easily from children. Now, there's a moment of panic when I'm presented with a child to treat who has a bacterial, viral, or fungal skin infection because I know how easily I catch it. It's like, "Ugh." I don't want to have that reaction to a child.

I worked through the glove issue with myself and the parents. I explained about universal precautions, and I wore gloves. I was able to help parents feel at ease, and it helped me feel at ease, too.

In the very beginning, I was angry at the parents. People who take drugs have a right to make that decision to destroy themselves, but they don't have the right to destroy their child. They leave the care of the child to others who have to go through so much emotional turmoil. I was very angry. Then I met some of the mothers, and they weren't the ogres that I thought they would be. They didn't deliberately cause the disease in the child. There are a number of mothers whose children I either see frequently in clinic or I'm treating. When the mother says, "I'm pregnant again," I feel like shouting, "I'm already treating two of your children. How could you do this?" I don't say that, but I feel like "here we go again." I feel like yelling, "Where's your responsibility? Where's your thought? How can you do this again?" Those are still some things that I need to work on.

Fortunately, these feelings don't spill over into my treatment. It's fairly easy for me to focus on the child. My focus on the mother is what she wants to know about her child. What is it that she wants from me? If you want me to show you ways of helping the children move or for you to manage them a little bit easier or to feed them a little bit better or to help you to understand what the disease is like in them, this is what I can do. How the parents got to these circumstances, what caused it, what their lifestyle is about, and what they're doing to either stay in it or get out of it really doesn't make that much difference to me.

I applaud the parents who are really working hard to change their lives. I try to be as supportive as possible. I guess I don't really see the ones who aren't taking some responsibility because those parents aren't getting their children in to see me. Many people on the team know much more about the family situation. I would rather be blind to the family situation, drug treatment program, family relationship problems, or all of those other issues. I only want to know their impact on my skills for the child and what I might be able to share with the parents.

Funerals and Grief

I don't cry about my patients now, although I did at one child's funeral. I don't cry easily about other people's plights or about problems associated with work. I feel more like digging in my heels and seeing what I can do. If there's stuff I can do, then I do it. If not, I let it go. I thought I'd be more affected by the deaths of the children. I made a decision not to go to all the funerals of all the children that I had been treating. Although I had a real close relationship with the first two or three groups of parents, there's no way that I could have maintained that intensity of emotion for the other families of the children. I went to the first three funerals. After that, I also changed locations so that I wasn't in the situation where I had as much contact with them.

The first baby funerals are a little hard to take, to see these kids in open caskets, dressed up in their christening or communion clothes, with stuffed animals around them. They're dead and gone, but I needed to be there for the parents to help them say goodbye. I needed to be there for me. That was an important part of accepting that AIDS is a fatal disease, and this is how it generally ends, at least given our current medical technology.

I initially needed to go through the whole grief process. Even though it really bothered me to see them laid out in the caskets, I needed to go through that. If I didn't do that, it would be different for me now. I almost forget that that's how it ends.

There are Limits: Lessons in Life

I originally wanted to identify the characteristics of children with HIV so that I'd know better how to intervene with physical therapy. I've improved with that and have been able to make some better treatment decisions. I know what physical therapy treatment can change and what it can't change, given the progressive nature of the disease. There have been times when I've been much more insistent on when a child should get treatment and times when it's not going to make any difference.

I periodically saw a child in a day care center where I consulted. She was also receiving early intervention services from another program, and she was discussed at a team meeting. One of the developmental specialists said, "She's not getting any better. She just seems to be getting

progressively worse, and she should be in a daily program
of physical therapy, occupational therapy, and speech." I
said, "There's no way that she's going to get that kind of
treatment, given the resources of early intervention and
availability of people. Even if you did that, it wouldn't
make any difference." One of the pediatricians asked how I
could say that. I told him, "The most important thing is that
we work with the people in day care so that she's moving
appropriately. That will prevent any contractures and defor-
mities, and we'll give the mom support when the child's
home so that she can manage her better. Having her in a
daily program of treatment isn't going to make any difference." I thought, "Have I opened my mouth now!"

One of the other pediatricians spoke up, "We're
dealing with a child who is probably in a relentlessly
progressive category of the disease. You're right. There's no
way that all the rehabilitation treatment in the world is
going to stop this disease. Nor do we have the medical technology to stop the progression of the disease. She's already
on AZT and on prophylactic respiratory pentamidine, which
is new with children. They've tried all the different things
that they could possibly try with her. She has a gastrostomy
tube (direct feeding to stomach) so she doesn't lose
weight." I added my two cents' worth: "I'm working with
her in feeding and movement, and she has speech, OT, and
PT in her other program. She's got loving people taking
care of her at the day care center. She has a mom who's
breaking her neck to try to get her to all the different things,
and we're not going to stop the disease. There's no way that
we're going to do that."

Being able to realize that there are limits and to feel
strongly enough to speak out were big steps for me. Back
when I was in a mode of thinking that physical therapy was

going to stop this miserable disease and prevent this child from dying, I was very unrealistic. Now, I'm a lot more realistic and say, "We can do the best that we can do, and that's all that we can do."

This experience has helped me crystallize some of the issues. New information comes out on a daily basis about this disease. Each child I see is a puzzle, and we have a limited time to solve the puzzle. I get so caught up in it. It's exciting to work in a field that's changing so rapidly. There's also the hope that we might make a difference. Maybe we can keep this child a little more functional while the medical community is finding ways to slow things down.

I have some specific feelings about putting children on AZT prophylactically almost at birth. You have a two-year window before the side effects of AZT become an issue. Would they live longer without the AZT? Would they live longer if you wait and put them on the AZT later? Would they do better if you didn't put them on AZT? Right now, the protocol is almost called for — prophylactic AZT, prophylactic gastrostomy tube. We have all these little kids who are getting fatter because they're on these nutritional feedings, but they're not moving any better.

Although AZT has some impact on changing muscle tone, I've got to work like mad trying to get the kids moving a little bit better in a situation where I'm not really seeing them for treatment. I can't just say to one of the developmental specialists that this child should be referred for treatment. She'll never get it because she lives in such and such an area. Will they treat kids with HIV? You can't tell them they have HIV. In some ways, the medical treatment has been good, but we need to be involved in a study where we're actually doing some comparisons of the efficacy of the treatment. Is it really making a difference in terms of value to the child?

I don't feel helpless. The danger, for me, is that one can easily become apathetic. "So I missed this one. So what?" I don't want to develop that attitude. I get frustrated, but if I can't do everything, I realize I can't carry the world of children with HIV infection on my shoulders. I've learned that I can share it with other people. It's not my responsibility to treat every single child that I see. That's a new realization for me! I'm still struggling with it.

In some ways, I've learned to accept humanness a bit better and to accept things that I can and can't change. The biggest change is in my attitude toward people who abuse drugs and the impact of that abuse on their families and children. I've become a lot more understanding and accepting of the factors that push people over the edge.

It's not a choice to get the disease. You can decide that you have to have your drugs, that you've got to be out on the street as a prostitute to get your drugs. You're not out there choosing to get a disease that's going to cause death.

I see these as stories. Everyone has a story. Sometimes, I really want to know. "How come you did that?" I once asked parents of a child who I treated. "Did you realize how sick this little girl was before you had adopted her? Were you aware of how sick this little girl was at three weeks or three months?" The mother said, "No, I thought she was fine." It's now eighteen months later. What are you going to do about it? That's my internal question, but I was quiet, waiting to see what else she would say. "Yes, now I see how sick she is, but that doesn't mean that we're going to give her up or give her back." Every time I treated this child, I never knew which family member was going to be coming for me to teach them what to do with her. I met everyone from the grandparents to the third generation. All came in to see what I was doing with this little girl so that they could do it at home, too.

I've never asked a natural mother who brought her child in for treatment, "What happened? Did you know what this was all about? Did you know how you got the disease? Do you know how your child got the disease?" I couldn't confront them with that. I listen to see if they are going to tell me the answers to my unasked questions: "Why did you bring the child for treatment? What is it you're looking for? How ill or how well are you? How are you coping with the disease? How are you coping with the child's disease? How's your family coping with it?" All those things eventually come out when you're treating someone three days a week and it's just you, the child, and the parents in a room together. They seem to open up more.

A Big Focus of My Life: AIDS and Me

Treating children with HIV has broadened my profession, and it's focused it toward clinical research. In fact, it has made me become a researcher whereas, previously, I had thought of myself as an administrator, teacher, and clinician. I've wanted to find out more about the disease and the disease process. I've been able to bring my knowledge and skill in dealing with children with neurological conditions to this new disease, and I've become a part of something that is on the forefront. It's kind of exciting to be part of something that is in the news almost on a daily basis. It's also a big focus of my life.

In some ways, working with kids with AIDS is a good antidote for dating circumstances. If I get into a hot and heavy dating situation, I can say, "Leave me alone. I'm an AIDS activist so I don't have casual sex with people." Maybe it gives me a legitimate excuse for scaring people off when I need to. I'm dating someone regularly now, but I'm still an educator. If I'm expected to talk to people about transmission of the disease, safe sex, and all of those issues, the least that I can do is practice what I preach. It's made me very cautious about what I teach other people. I don't want to put it under the rug, saying, "That happens to other people."

Being involved with the disease on a daily basis, I'm also aware of practicing safe sex. Are you practicing the same things that you tell other people they should? Can you hold the same standards for yourself that you hold for other people? It makes me look at the standards that I hold other people to and ask myself, "Am I doing that?"

I don't buy into that "innocent victim" stuff. People don't realize the potential of this disease. Their behavior makes a difference in whether they get it or don't. It's a disease that no one knew was coming. All of a sudden it was here, and everyone was a victim of this disease. Some got caught, and some didn't. Even adults didn't have a choice. They didn't know what they were up against until they got it.

When I was living in England, I had a friend who had developed AIDS, and for a long time, he denied that he had the disease. He talked about how he picked up an infection when he was doing a show in Africa. "Everyone thinks that I have AIDS, and they're absolutely wrong. I don't." I'd never confront him with it and say, "You know, you probably do." There was a time when he had gotten ill and recovered. A lot of people were shunning him. "Oh, yes, he's a hairdresser. He's got AIDS. Everybody knows that." By then, I had moved away from England. On a return visit, he asked me, "When are you coming to dinner?" He told me, "People don't invite me to dinner anymore." I was dumbfounded. "What do you mean they don't invite you to dinner anymore? That's stupid." He eventually died of the disease. My only regret was that I didn't get back to see him in London as he became more ill.

I felt terribly saddened that I didn't learn about his death until weeks afterward because I think I would have gone over to England to go to his funeral. I would have seen his mom and dad and been able to be with them because I knew a lot about the stigma they were dealing with. I wanted them to know that I didn't feel that way. I don't care whether he had the disease or not, he was still one of the most delightful people and certainly the best hairdresser I ever had in my life. What a terrible waste of talent that he's gone.

Chapter Ten

Debbie: Vulnerability and the Meaning of Life

Doing this work has made me re-examine a number of things in my life, such as my friendships and relationships. I've had to decide what and who are important to me. I've struggled over the past years, feeling very isolated.

Debbie is a forty-three-year-old white woman who is heterosexual. A nurse for twenty years, she has worked with AIDS patients for five years, treating more than one hundred AIDS patients in the past year in a long-term care facility.

Unlike a medical-surgical nurse, the picture that frequently comes to mind when people think of a nurse, Debbie is a psychiatric nurse. She specializes in the care and treatment of mental health rather than physical health. Working with people with AIDS, she addresses areas of psychiatric problems, dementia, suicidal thoughts and actions, to name a few. Part of her job is to work with staff members to raise their awareness of these concerns and their impact on patient care. She also serves as a facilitator of a nurses' support group to discuss how they cope with working with these patients.

Debbie is not married and has no significant other. Her friends and family don't want to hear about her work, and as a group facilitator, she's not in a position to share her problems with the others.

At times, she feels completely burned out and needs more frequent vacations in this job than in any other she has had. She exercises to work off her day. She also goes to therapy to discuss several issues, including her work.

Because more than two hundred patients have died in the past four years, Debbie has been reflecting on her own vulnerability and the meaning of life. She chose this work with her eyes wide open, knowing death would be a part of it. Still, it has a major impact on her.

Debbie is trying to value her life to a larger degree and experience it more fully. Knowing that she should enjoy life doesn't make it happen. She asks herself hard life questions: Why don't I feel better? Why don't I appreciate my life more? What do I need to change?

Choices and Support

I came into this work by choice rather than being assigned to this unit. The connection between the medical and psychiatric problems attracted me. People were afraid of AIDS, yet I gravitated toward it. My first year in graduate school, I worked in a psychiatric facility, and we had a number of seriously ill AIDS patients. At some point during that year, I decided that I really wanted to continue working with these patients. I talked with people in my graduate program and got a placement where there were many AIDS patients. I knew this unit was being established and kept my ears open to see if they would be looking for a psychiatric nurse. It was clearly a time that I was looking for some changes and trying to do things differently.

When I started in AIDS work, it wasn't brand new, but I still felt on the cutting edge. I had worked with psychiatric inpatients for a long time. I feel more exhilarated now. Being more involved in a medical illness, doing more consultation, and trying to figure out what's going on at any given time is challenging. Trying to fathom whether a patient is delirious, demented, or depressed is fun. I feel like a detective.

I enjoy teaching the staff, but I get frustrated when I feel like I'm working with people who either are not capable or don't want to learn. When I'm teaching a nurse, and she or he really starts getting it, I love that — that's the most exhilarating thing.

My family couldn't understand why I was interested in psychiatric nursing. Because they never understood that, I also never expected them to understand my wanting to work with AIDS patients.

The hard thing is my friends' lack of support. On the surface, they seem interested and proud of my work, but they don't want to hear about it. There's a lot of lip service. If I'm down, they ask why I'm still doing it. It's very hard sometimes to try to convey to people what it's really like. They might tell me something about a person with AIDS, saying, "Isn't this horrible?" I want to scream, "It's no big deal. I hear worse every day."

Intimate Moments

Working with people with AIDS is challenging and has pushed me in a number of ways. At different times, it's been very exhilarating, very stressful, and very depressing. It's also been very, very sad. It's been filled with surprises and changes, which is important to me because I tend to get bored easily. Doing this work, I've had some of the most intimate moments in my life.

I've been surprised at how close I've gotten to some of the people here. During my first two years here, I worked with a lot of prisoners. At that time, state policy said that once a patient was diagnosed with AIDS, he went to the hospital and stayed there until he either died or was released from prison. Several of us on the staff developed extremely intense relationships with those patients. We saw them every day for years. That's more than I see my family.

I remember a guy who was twenty-three when he was diagnosed. He was kind of a young punk in a very endearing way. He would get very angry and occasionally show up here drunk or high on drugs. He was threatening and scary to some people. I had seen him at his most vulnerable when he was first diagnosed with AIDS. That tends to cut through so much garbage. He was in a lot of pain toward the end and was already on very high levels of medication. Every day during his last week, the physician assistant and I would start and end our day with him. We'd go in to see him and clean him up, which was not a part of either of our jobs, and touch and hold him. He was still alert enough to clearly know that we were there with him. You don't have that kind of intimacy with a lot of people. It was a pretty incredible experience. It really helped me finish things in a very concrete way.

When someone's dying, I usually sit and talk with them. Touching becomes very important to me, being able to hold people and be caring. This has been unique for me. I've been a psychiatric nurse for a long time, and touching is not a normal part of what I do with patients. Touching the patient is a big difference in working with people with HIV. I've had to re-evaluate the normal boundaries that I've had with patients without HIV.

When I met one of my first patients with AIDS, I held out my hand to shake his. He told me that his physician put on a gown, gloves, mask, and a mask over his stethoscope every time he touched him. Extending my hand was very important to him. There are so many ways in which touch is vital with these people.

I needed to figure out whether I was touching people for my own need or because it was helpful for them. That's not always easy for me to figure out. My touch conveys that I want to be there with them. I can listen. Somehow, words don't seem to always work. There's a certain gentleness that people sometimes need and don't often get. Most nurses are very task-oriented and busy. Sometimes, touching is a way to slow down and say, "I'm here just for you, not to give you pills or do this procedure or change your bed."

Sadness and Endings

During my first year here, I had gotten close to people. It was very sad for me when I lost them. I worked with one man for almost a year, and we initially had a good, solid relationship. He used the time with me to deal with a lot of anger and get support. Then something went wrong, and I never totally figured it out. He was requiring lots of pain medication and would often be very sedated. I tried to talk to him about it, and he heard that as an attack. He was so angry with me that he stopped talking to me for about a month. I tried everything I knew, but he continued to refuse to talk to me. As he deteriorated, we connected again a little, but by then, he was somewhat demented and affected by the medication. We never really finished our business. It was hard and made me feel very sad.

Perhaps he thought I betrayed him. Before I brought up the medication issue, he told me that he knew I was there to listen to him and hear his story. Maybe he thought that I had stepped outside of what he wanted the relationship to be. It was very sad that we couldn't talk about it. I felt cheated that I couldn't get closure in the relationship, frustrated that I couldn't make things right.

This experience was probably the most painful as well as the saddest for me. I cried hard after that. I knew when I left work, the day he died, that he wasn't going to make it through the night. I had spent a lot of time with him that afternoon. He also had an AIDS buddy with whom I worked. I called the buddy later in the evening, and he said to me, "He just died." It was just like, "Yeow!" It felt really weird to be on the phone as this was happening. That's how close I felt to him. Fortunately, I don't get that involved with very many people.

I'm fairly comfortable feeling sad and letting myself cry when I need to. I get close to certain individuals, and I've cried with some patients. I cry when patients with whom I'm close die, but I usually cry with other people. I don't generally go home and cry alone.

I never go to funerals, but I attend every single hospital memorial service. I helped initiate these services and asked the hospital chaplain to do them rather than try to do them myself. He expects me to be there and wants and needs a little direction. A big part of my job is dealing with the nursing staff. I need to be a role model for them by attending the memorial services and trying to deal with feelings on work time. Many people here do go to funerals, which concerns me. Some people make AIDS their life and go to the funeral of every patient who dies on this unit. It's not healthy. By taking a leadership role in organizing on-the-job memorial services, I'm taking care of business, although it's not easy.

A Veteran Amidst Turnover

People don't do this work for a long period of time. When I started here, the AIDS unit had been open for seven months, and we were already experiencing the first massive turnover in the nursing staff. There was another turnover in less than a year. Now we have a more stable team of nurses. Although we try to be an interdisciplinary team, there has always been a separation. There is the nursing staff and then there is another group that consists of the social worker, the psychiatrist, the medical director, a nurse practitioner, a physician assistant, and me. This second group has really been my peer group, and a number of those people have left the unit in the last year.

Having been a pioneer, I feel like a veteran. The turnover in the non-nursing group is significant because that group has more input into new policies and directions. Over the last three or four months, some have wanted to implement changes, without understanding why a particular idea or policy was in existence. I felt like a history bearer, explaining why something was important. The process was disturbing because it felt like things have changed so much.

The AIDS unit has been a little haven within this totally crazy state system. We have demanded and gotten away with a higher expectation of patient care on this unit than in the rest of the hospital. People have resisted many attempts to lower our level of care. I'm worried that when the rest of the old-timers leave, everything we've worked for will collapse.

I support the nurses as part of my job but have trouble getting support for myself. The first year I was here was horrible because I didn't know anybody. I was very cautious who I shared things with because of my role. There was another psychiatric nurse in the hospital who was a geriatric clinical specialist, and it took a while to develop a relationship with her. I eventually did get support from her. The psychiatrist who I worked with the first year was terrible, and we didn't get along. After she left, her replacement was magnificent and was one of my main sources of support until he left a little over a year ago. The social worker on this unit became a very strong source of support, but she also left about a year ago. There's another new psychiatric medical specialist on the TB unit, and she and I are doing peer support.

I think there are two nurses who have been here as long or longer than I have. The medical director started a couple of weeks after I did, and the physician assistant has been here since the opening. We're the old-timers. There has been a massive change.

On the Road to Burnout

I feel very isolated. AIDS isn't something people want to discuss. At times, it's been a major part of my life. There are frequently very intense, emotional experiences that people have here. When you go home and can't say anything about them to your spouse and your best friend, that's a problem.

I feel absolutely burned out at times. Physical exercise, wearing myself out physically, has become much more important to me. I've quit smoking since I've been here so the exercise, I think, in some ways is a replacement for that. I've gotten into therapy since I've been here for a combination of issues, including my work. I try to plan frequent vacations and try to have some idea of when and what my next vacation is before the present one ends. That has been very important to me since my first year here. If I don't have a vacation or at least longer than a three-day weekend every three to four months, I'm not in good shape.

This is the first job I've needed that much time off. In other jobs, I've managed to go for six months to a year without a vacation, without feeling like I was getting burned out. I can't do that in this job. It's good to know that. There are still times when I don't catch it fast enough.

There are lots of frustrations here. We sometimes don't attract high level staff. There are a lot of psychosocial issues in dealing with AIDS. I work with staff members on issues like how to deal with another human being or how to be a professional. I shouldn't have to deal with someone screaming at patients, but I do, over and over again. Working in this place is like working in the United Nations. There are so many cultural groups and many clashes among different cultures. In some ways, it's been eye-opening and fun, but it's frustrating, too.

I often feel least effective with others on the staff. I have been frustrated and lost my patience more times than I would like to admit. Psychiatric care is frequently not valued as much as physical care. Many patients on this unit have needed one-to-one supervision because they're confused, wandering, or suicidal. There have been many episodes where staff members don't understand the importance of this and walk away. I've talked about it from a legal point of view. I've talked about it from a liability point of view. I've talked about it from the patients' safety point of view. I've talked about the dynamics until I finally screamed. Part of my frustration is that I'm not capable of changing others' attitudes. Direction has to come from the administrators, who often seem not to value what we do either. There's tremendous pressure because of staffing and money problems. I keep hearing, "Why is this person still on one-to-one? When are you going to take him off?" When he's not suicidal anymore, we'll take him off precautions.

Staff members sometimes scream at patients, and I sometimes scream at the staff. I'm not effective when I scream. Others may get totally irritated with patients, but I don't. I get totally irritated with the staff.

There have been staffing changes over time. There have also been changes in our patient population. At one time, I felt like the token straight person here. That's not true anymore. When I first started on this unit, most patients were primarily gay men. Now, they are primarily drug users, black and Hispanic men mostly. We usually have only one woman at a time. Most people's risk category is IV drug use. Sometimes we get partners of IV drug users and

an occasional hemophiliac. It's not easy to develop a relationship with some of these people.

I feel very little fear. That's not to say that I don't
have twinges of some irrational fear at times. I'm almost at
no risk. I've touched people, but I don't have contact with
body fluids very often. I'm at a bigger risk for TB. TB is a
big issue with AIDS patients. Sometimes I worry about that.

Life's Lessons on the AIDS
Roller Coaster

When I started working with people with AIDS, I
anticipated that I was going to be learning a lot and dealing
with a number of personal issues. It's hard to face this many
dying people without looking at your own vulnerability. It
boggles my mind that more than two hundred people have
died here in the last four years. That's not something you
can experience without trying to think about what life
means and what it's all about. By choosing to do this work,
I am choosing to deal with those issues. I'm not sorry that I
have!

I think everybody is pretty innocent about getting
AIDS. Very few people go out there and shoot drugs in their
arms and think they're going to get AIDS. I think all of us
take risks in life and don't necessarily think about the
consequences. The desire for drugs is so overwhelming for
most of these people that exposing themselves to AIDS is
just a minor issue.

One patient was both interesting and hard for me to
work with. He had a long psychiatric history with major
suicide attempts. He actually told us that he went out trying
to get AIDS as a way to kill himself. One day he'd be on

suicide watch, and the next day he'd be very physically ill, fighting hard to stay alive. It feels like a roller coaster here.

There are a lot of roller coasters with this disease. People can get very ill very quickly. I've been with people and seen stark changes over the course of an hour. At the beginning of the hour, they're okay, and by the end of the hour, they're shivering, have a temperature of 105 and are on their way to a serious medical illness. It's pretty weird to watch all that in one hour. I say good-bye to people, and they reappear six months later. There's also a tremendous amount of fluctuation with the dementia for people, and that's hard to take. I was on a roller coaster a lot of times during my first year or so. I would drive to work wondering, what are we confronting today?

Doing this work has had a major impact on what I want out of life. It's forcing me to look at life in a way I haven't done before. I continue struggling with its importance. The lesson to be learned here is to really enjoy life while you have it. I see people every day who wish that they could go back in time and have moments to live over again or wish they could have done things differently. I look at nice things in my life and wonder why I don't appreciate life more. How come it doesn't feel better? What do I need to do to change that? That's the most crucial point and personal challenge that I get from dealing with people who have AIDS.

As I've gained experience and gotten older, I'm better able to anticipate some of the problems I'm walking into and walk in with a clearer vision. I'm a little better prepared to deal with the sadness. Part of my personal style of coping is to come up with worst-case scenarios as a way to prepare myself for something to happen. I'm more cynical than I used to be, and I'm not happy about that. I would like that to change. Ten years ago, I probably would have thought twice before saying a lot of what I say now.

I've learned a lot about myself, and I don't like everything I see. I'm not very patient, and that has been a big thing for me to see. I've also looked at how being in a helping role has been such a big part of my life. It's not something new to me, but I'm thinking about it much more seriously now.

I have lower expectations of patients than I used to have. That probably takes some pressure off them. I have higher expectations of other staff members, but I would do well to lower those expectations. If I lower them too much, though, what would be left? It's a matter of principle with me.

Working in the state system has been a real eye-opener. It's a dysfunctional system. You can only stay so long without being gravely affected by it. People come into work not knowing if their unit, or the hospital, is going to remain open. We don't know if we're going to be laid off or bumped in our positions. This is my furlough day — I'm working for free today. AIDS patients need care regardless of state budgets!

This work is unique for me. It's different from any other nursing I've done. I may be reaching a point where I can't do this a whole lot longer, though. I don't think it's healthy for me to do this very much longer. It's been five years. That's a good chunk of time. Maybe I'll take a break and return, although I haven't seen many people return.

Chapter Eleven

Mark: Discovering Value
Judgments and Biases

When you're dealing with people who have a scientific background, you'd like to think that they would respond to issues with scientific thinking. That hasn't happened across the board in dentistry and medicine.

Mark is a fifty-three-year-old, white, heterosexual man who works as a dental practitioner. An oral-maxillofacial surgeon, he has twenty-six years of experience in his field, five with people with AIDS, and has treated twenty-five people with AIDS in the past year in his private practice.

Unlike a general dentist, who may treat patients throughout their lives, he sees patients on a short-term basis, treating them in hospital emergency rooms, surgical suites, and his private office. His patients are usually in pain and have many kinds of oral surgical problems, such as broken jaws.

Married, with grown children, Mark only recently realized that he grew up with values and beliefs that made him very judgmental and prejudiced. The values of his family, friends, ethnic group, and religious training contributed to his point of view, making it difficult for him to accept a person for what he or she is. He was repulsed listening to a gay man talk about sharing life with his partner. Intellectually, he considered himself open-minded and tolerant, yet he thought homosexual behavior and the people were abnormal. As he allows himself to listen to more people, he understands more about others.

Although he feels good about treating all patients equally, including those who are HIV-positive, he's learning some hard lessons about himself.

Accepting Patients After They've Been Rejected by Others

There have been occasions when HIV-positive individuals have been referred to us by medical colleagues who know that we treat all people. Those patients may have been turned away at one or more offices and often are in severe pain. They may have been in pain for days. The HIV-positive individuals may have to go through a number of telephone calls and embarrassing situations and rejections before they're able to find a health care worker who is willing to take care of their needs.

Patients are referred to us by medical colleagues rather than dental colleagues. Internists who see many HIV-positive individuals will get complaints when a patient has been turned away at a particular dental office. All of the referrals that we get are because of the nature of the surgery that needs to be done. Other physicians know they can call here and secure an appointment. I'm aware of dental practitioners who refuse to take on these patients, but I can't remember a situation where a dentist specifically called and said, "I'm not going to take care of this patient. I want you to take care of him because he's HIV-positive."

We had a significant problem of access to dental care in this state, and I'm sure that other states have similar situations. We developed a program to get the names of dentists who would volunteer to be on a list — "Yes, I will take care of HIV-positive individuals." I was opposed to that concept because it doesn't foster treating everyone who comes into our office. It's important that the practice of dentistry and medicine respond to the needs of those who can knock on their door or call them on the telephone. That's the way things are supposed to be done.

In the program initiated by the state AIDS project, the health department, and the state dental association, we could receive a telephone call from an HIV-positive individual or from a physician who wanted to refer an HIV-positive person. The protocol was that the HIV-positive individual could choose the dentist that he or she would like to go to, as they would normally choose from the phone book. They would then call that dentist and ask for an appointment. We knew that there would be another problem — some dental offices don't take Medicaid or welfare.

We advised these people to be up front and tell the dentist that they were on Medicaid or welfare when they secured the appointment. We put together a letter to send to the dentist once the patient got the appointment. The letter informed the dentist that there would be an HIV-positive patient, no names involved, who would be coming to the office for an appointment. The letter also explained that, as an agency, we would like to help the dentist with infection-control measures in the office. If they had any questions, they could call us, and the health department would send someone in. The dental association had educational tapes available to teach proper infection-control measures. If the patient was rejected, we asked the individual to let us know who the dentist was. Again, not to police the dentist. Our group would call the dentist, state our knowledge that the practitioner had turned away a person because of HIV-positive status, and inquire if there was anything that their colleagues, the dental association, or the health department could do to help them get over this hurdle.

Obviously, it was an uphill battle because AIDS is a very emotional issue. There are emotional overtones that place value judgments on people because of their lifestyles. We feel we've made some progress because the people from the state AIDS project and those physicians who have seen many HIV-positive patients now receive fewer complaints from their patients and clients that they cannot access dental care. We've also conducted statewide continuing education programs, trying to educate the dentist, the dental hygienist, and the dental assistant. That's something. We'll probably continue these programs on a yearly basis.

There have been cases that went to the Human Rights Commission. We have a law in this state prohibiting refusals to treat on the basis of HIV-positive status or even the assumption that the person might be gay, HIV-positive, or a drug abuser. The law should have curtailed many of these issues from developing. A letter went to all members of the American Dental Association telling them that even though they had malpractice insurance, there would be consequences if they were brought to task in a court of law or before the Human Rights Commission because they had turned away an HIV-positive person.

Still there are problems. Usually, it's lack of education and understanding. The dentist may be willing, but the hygienist may say, "If you treat an HIV-positive patient, I'm going to leave the practice." Sometimes, it's the opposite. The hygienist, dental assistant, or the young ladies at the desk are willing to treat, but the dentist doesn't want to. It becomes a matter of trying to educate everyone. When we had our conference in November, we invited all employees from the office and had a good turnout of hygienists and assistants along with dentists.

I don't really think of people with AIDS as different patients. I think of them as patients that I would normally be treating in the office. I try not to pigeonhole people. People don't like to be treated differently because of their handicaps, which includes having an infectious disease. People who are HIV-positive seem to appreciate that I treat them as I would anyone else. I take care of their needs and don't make any particular reference to their infectious disease. I consider that rewarding.

I like to conduct my practice in an appropriate fashion for someone who wants to serve the public as a health care professional. I think that's part of our responsibility. Some individuals within my profession don't view it this way. They view their practice as one where they can pick and choose who they want to treat. In my specialty of oral-maxillofacial surgery, we see patients in pain all the time. We see patients in accident rooms where we deal with cracked jaws and a variety of surgical problems. Our cases are different from the general practitioner's, who takes care of gums or teeth. He may not view things the same way that I do.

Of Risks and Icebergs

One of the things that has been stressed in education with dental health care workers is that the person may be HIV-positive and not even know it. When you treat that patient, you run the same risk as with the person who indicates that he or she is HIV-positive or has full-blown AIDS. People have this misconception that the only ones they have to worry about are the ones who come in and say, "Yes, I'm HIV-positive."

The American Dental Association has tried to stress infection control. Universal precautions are for everyone. You can't conduct a practice today in which you can isolate those who might be infectious. It's fairly common knowledge that the ones who will tell you they are HIV-positive are the very top peak of an iceberg, and there are large numbers of people underneath the water. No one knows how deep that water is, because of the number of people who may be infected and don't know it. Initially, it was thought that those infected were all gay men, and that's not the scenario we see today. Hemophiliacs, heterosexuals, health care workers, and others have been involved. The risk comes with the responsibility of doing the work that I do. A person who is a steel worker and works on bridges understands that you run the risk of falling off the bridge. A police officer runs the risk of being hurt on his job.

Early in this epidemic, statements from the American Dental Association and the American Medical Association said that when we entered a room with a person who was HIV-positive, we were to wear a lot of protective garments — a cap, mask, a garment that would cover us down to our wrists, shoe covers, etc. People thought that it was going to be impossible to see known AIDS or HIV-positive patients in the office because donning protective garments isn't the normal thing one does in general practice. To complicate matters, we'd have to decontaminate the room afterward. It threw a tremendous scare into a lot of people.

It was so erroneous and overplayed that, to this day, there are still some people who think that way. They give the impression that they understand the concept of what one needs to do to treat patients. Yet, if I ask them, "What do you do when you treat an AIDS patient?" they'll say, "When I treat someone who I know has AIDS, I'll put double gloves on and wear a couple of extra garments. I'll do something special with the instruments and the room."

Then I ask, "What do you do with the person who you don't know is HIV-positive or they don't know that they're HIV-positive but are just as infected?" That's a stumbling block because they categorize the person with AIDS as being totally different, needing to be treated differently. That's a difficult hurdle to overcome because the initial information made a lasting impression.

The fact that the hepatitis virus has been around for a long time can give a dental or medical practitioner a sense of what this issue of HIV is all about. We have all known about the hepatitis virus, and the AMA and ADA have encouraged their practitioners to secure the hepatitis vaccine. If anyone is practicing dentistry or medicine, including dentists, dental hygienists, and assistants, they should get the vaccine. The compliance for having the vaccine on hand was slow in rising, it was 25 percent or 30 percent at one time. It's actually better in dentistry than it is in medicine now. I think that we're up to 70 percent or 75 percent after many, many years.

Why are there still practitioners out there who don't avail themselves of the hepatitis vaccine? The hepatitis virus is much more infectious. For some, the issue is monetary. It costs $100 or $200. They don't want to spend that, and they certainly don't want to spend it on one, two, or ten employees. Some of these folks are unreachable. Even sitting with them, on a one-to-one basis, we can't convince them that it's impossible to continue to practice dentistry without ever seeing an HIV-positive individual. There's no such thing as an isolated cubicle in the office.

Take the orthodontists. As a group, orthodontists classically feel that they're treating people where they run the least risk. They think that they don't run a risk because they treat teenagers and youngsters. Very few orthodontists wear gloves, and they don't use masks. They don't worry about the little wire clippings that come off. They don't view them as "sharps," and they should be dealt with as "sharps." I've spoken to orthodontic groups and told them about this. Today, compared to fifty years ago, more orthodontists are treating adults and promiscuous teenagers. There may be many out there who are HIV-positive, and you don't even know, because it may take eight to ten years before they begin to show any AIDS-type symptoms.

Hostility and Secrets

When I deal with an individual who has been turned away many times at some other office or offices, I try to be as cordial and friendly as I would with any other patient. Despite that, there's often hostility on the patient's part. I don't have any control over that. He or she has been discriminated against or treated poorly and views me as the same kind of health care worker, as though I'm no better than the next guy down the street. I get frustrated.

In our type of practice, we see most of our patients only one time, unlike in a general practitioner's office, where he may have the patient for a lifetime. Someone comes in here with a toothache or a broken jaw, and we take care of it. We may see them once or twice, and then they're gone. It's hard to sit down and try to turn that person's viewpoint of dentistry around. All I can do is try to be caring.

We had a young man a couple of years ago who we saw off and on for a while. We only found out he was HIV-positive after he'd been here a number of times, and we had done several procedures on him. He always gave the impression that no matter what was done, there was no way that we could do enough for him. It was either that the people downstairs were rude, or when he would call in the middle of the night the answering service would be rude, or the folks who answered the phone for the answering service were rude. He was a difficult person to please. When I found out that he was HIV-positive, I remember asking him if I could speak with him privately. I had my assistants leave the room and close the door, and I told him that I knew that he was HIV-positive. He had presented to the accident room at the local hospital and was having a bleeding situation from some recent oral surgery that we did on him. The emergency room physician knew that I'd been treating him and wanted to make me aware of the fact that the man was HIV-positive. His bleeding was a related problem because his platelet count was affected. The physician wasn't trying to disclose anything but was trying to help me in treating the patient.

Trying to get him to understand that it was important to me as a practitioner to know that he was HIV-positive was almost impossible. I wasn't placing a value judgment on him. I was trying to be able to take care of his needs. I told him that I could understand, but I encouraged him to tell others in the future. He might be in a situation where someone was trying to diagnose a symptom or a sign and couldn't because he didn't know that the man was HIV-positive. It's like a diabetic having a problem, and someone asking, "Do you have diabetes?" "No, I'm not diabetic." Unless you run some tests on the individual, you're not going to know what you're dealing with. He told me that every time he indicated that he was HIV-positive, he was turned away.

That's a common story I hear from HIV-positive people. They don't want to disclose any more because they've been turned away too many times. There was a little hostility between some of the young ladies in the office and this individual only because he was very rude and offensive. When they knew that he had failed to disclose that he was HIV-positive, they were really annoyed. Immediately, he sensed friction, and there was nothing that we could do to please him.

We continued to treat him. One day, someone came in and told me that they had seen in the paper that he had died. He was probably in his twenties, and we were all upset. I can understand how he could become angry at the world and view people as antagonistic and threatening.

Hard Lessons to Learn

I recently attended an excellent conference. They had about a half-dozen HIV-positive people on a panel with clinicians, physicians, and oral pathologists. The audience was dentists, physicians, and health care workers. One panelist was gay, one a drug abuser, one a nurse who contracted the HIV virus while working.

The conference brought up more for me than I imagined. I grew up with certain value judgments. You can't help that, you're a product of your environment at home, your upbringing, your religious training, and your ethnic background. Your values get passed along from your parents and peers as you grow and mature. When you confront someone who views things differently, like sexual preference or drug abuse, it can be a difficult emotional task to try to overlook the differences. It's hard just to evaluate the person as a person.

There was a young lady on the panel who came in with a black leather jacket and spiked up hair. A conservative individual with my values would look at her and immediately think that this is a hippie problem. Her speaking mannerisms showed a sense of real hostility toward the folks in the audience, and she admitted that. We had a discussion about this, but it was hard for me to allow her to speak and express her feelings and values. I tried to listen to her viewpoints to see if they had some merit. Of all the people there, I had the toughest time getting over that hurdle with her, and I told her that. She was very abrupt and ill-mannered.

One evening, she and her boyfriend, who also wore a motorcycle jacket, gave a talk about what they were doing with ACT UP, what they were trying to do in Washington for women who are HIV-positive, and all the obstacles they've had to overcome. She was very abrupt, but her boyfriend was well-spoken. They both had a terrific message. These kids really put in a lot of time. They've been in jail a number of times because they were involved with ACT UP. Their ultimate goal was to help a certain group of people, and they felt that the government made it difficult for them to be able to achieve their objectives. I could sympathize with them, and I told her. Initially, I was so turned off by her, but after hearing all that she had to say that evening, I was really impressed with what she was trying to do.

I think she also felt hostility toward me initially, and toward others in the audience who were straight — that was her term, straight. She assumed that we were against her because she was HIV-positive and because of her dress. She indicated that she came away feeling differently about us, too. It was a growing experience for her having to deal with straight people. She could better understand that they also had some good values and feelings to express. I suggested that ACT UP shouldn't be quite so rude with their movement. She said that they would never get anywhere if they weren't. After hearing their story, I guess she was probably right. They've had to really push and shove and be abusive, be vocal and discourteous to get where they are. I think they've made big strides.

As much as I'd like to think that I'm very broad-minded in accepting all people, I've learned that I still have some prejudices that are hard to get over. I remember sitting next to one of the gay men at dinner during this conference. He was talking about his lover and sharing things with his lover. I found that difficult because that's not a norm for me. I was repulsed. With my upbringing, it's difficult to evaluate the person as a person and see what they have to offer.

The conference leaders showed a movie about the AIDS quilt project. It's very emotional and educational, something that every citizen should see. It was terrific. They go through the lives of a half-dozen people who are represented on the quilt, and one of them was this fellow I sat with at dinner. It's hard to understand how one man can feel this kind of love for another man. That was tough for me to watch, sitting there and thinking about how unnatural that seemed to me. It was abnormal. I don't know that it made me feel uncomfortable as much as it made me think about how I was responding. This was a learning process. I probably am more accepting of those people today than I was before.

You could go to a prison and take care of patients and try not to view them as criminals, but simply as other people. That's tough. As much as a person may say, "I just view them as another person," I still view them as a criminal. What did they do? Did they kill their mother? Some psychologist would probably tell you that there were some things you could never change, but it's important, if we're practicing medicine or dentistry, to overlook all those things when we're trying to treat someone.

Ethics is a universal problem that our society is dealing with. People think in terms of "me." "I decide who I treat. Don't tell me who I should treat. It's not my responsibility to treat someone who I think has an infectious disease or because they're on welfare. I don't treat those folks. I treat who I want to treat." That mentality is a product of our society.

Many practitioners say, "I don't want to ruin my practice. If my patients knew that I treated HIV-positive and AIDS patients, my practice would be ruined." That's an absolutely asinine statement. As a matter of fact, there's a dentist I know who has a sign in his waiting room indicating, "We treat HIV-positive patients. We treat all patients who come to our office, and we use infection control measures for all patients." He has a booming practice.

People have asked me, "Aren't you concerned?" I'm not, because I think it's my obligation. We have a very large practice, and we've been very successful. We treat all people who come in. There are certainly some people who might not go to an office because there was an HIV-positive or AIDS patient. If that were generally true, though, why hasn't it affected our practice?

Chapter Twelve

Putting It All Together: What It's Like to Work with People with AIDS

I've been very pleasantly surprised to see that I have a lot more in common with the patients than most people like to acknowledge.

Marlene, physician

We've listened to the heartfelt stories of nurses, physical therapists, a physician, a dental surgeon, and social workers who work with people with AIDS. As we've seen, several common themes emerge from their individual experiences:

- the intensity of their feelings
- dealing with the meaning of loss and death
- personal and professional growth issues, and
- the significance of their work.

Riding the Roller Coaster:
The Intensity of Feelings

As these health workers develop intimacy with people who they ordinarily would not under other circumstances, they experience a range of emotions. The emotions don't necessarily surprise them, but the intensity of these feelings is profound. Despite mentions of happiness and fun, the generic emotions are sadness and pain. Surprisingly, only one caregiver uses the word "depressing." Equally surprising, no one speaks about empathy, although there seem to be empathic connections between the caregivers and the patients. They talk candidly about their anger and situations in which they feel ineffective in their professional roles.

Health professionals experience anger when their efforts don't improve clients' lives and when community systems fail to adequately meet the multiple needs of the people with AIDS. They feel annoyed at patients when they're self-destructive and don't follow recommended treatment and behavior. They also get distressed when patients act irresponsibly and risk transmitting the virus to sexual partners and children.

Health workers are angry with parents and siblings who reject family members because of their lifestyles. They're annoyed when families don't take advantage of support services. Some are mad at colleagues who disregard safety issues. And finally, they're at odds with themselves when they lose their tempers or are careless with infection-control procedures.

Professionals feel frustrated by the difficulty of arranging community services for patients, limitations on their time, and hostile, angry patients. This is especially true when they work hard, feel they should do even more, and care about the patients. Burnout is on the minds of health care professionals working with people with AIDS. Steve is weary of being a cheerleader, trying to motivate people to change their high risk behavior. Other caregivers have difficulty setting boundaries and recognizing their limitations. Marlene feels drained by the endless needs of the patients and is unable to say no to them. Kim must remind herself to work only her eight-hour shift.

Interestingly, those few professionals who claim that they don't feel burned out initiated the conversation on the subject. Jessie adds the word "yet." Laura notes that she frequently changes jobs, ending her employment before burnout can develop.

The awful reality of patient decline and death is exhausting, and most of the professionals recognize that their coping mechanisms and defenses often are inadequate to combat negative emotions. Subsequently, these feelings of futility contribute to burnout. Caregivers must deal with continually changing information. Patients experience often dramatic fluctuations because of the volatile nature of their illness. Competent care doesn't always mean a patient will improve. This can shake one's professional confidence if backsliding occurs frequently. Reflecting upon the positive accomplishments — improved health and functioning, discharges to home, and available housing — becomes more than a survival skill. It almost becomes a personal mantra and a locker room pep talk to rejuvenate their energies, interests, and confidence.

Working within a state system notorious for budget reductions, understaffing, and overwork seems to promote burnout and is a source of frustration and occupational stress. Debbie thinks that the state system is dysfunctional and has a negative impact on its employees. Lack of support on the job, such as vacation coverage and adequate staffing, often contributes to an employee's lowered energy and coping strategies. Dennis says he sometimes feels too exhausted to spend time with patients. Marlene claims that even though the number of patients has increased over the years, the staff has not. It's noteworthy that only the public health workers brought up these points. Because many people with AIDS are treated in state facilities, this trend does not bode well for recruiting and keeping health professionals who care for them.

Although certain emotions are uniquely experienced by some of the health care professionals, sadness is universally shared. Caregivers struggle with the sorrow of working with patients whose course is marked by decline and death. They're saddened by the young age of the patients, their prognosis, and downward progression. Elaine describes a knee-jerk response of sadness for the young age of the people whom she treats.

Knowing that connections with patients, with whom health workers have long-term relationships, will ultimately end with the patients' death, naturally produces sorrow. Being a bystander watching the interruption and brevity of predominantly young lives and seeing their health begin to fail as they near death is, of course, emotionally draining. Friendships are often developed, and the losses have great impact on the professionals. Although experience and maturity strengthen the caregivers and ease the impact, the sorrow never fully leaves. Comfortable with feeling their grief, many caregivers sometimes allow themselves to cry about the frustration or injustice of people's circumstances. Some shed tears at work, in the car, or at home. Others never cry.

Coping with pain and sustaining life are central issues to a health care career. If parts of these core issues are repeatedly unsuccessful, the caregivers feel the anguish. As Elaine realizes, death from AIDS is not a "once in a blue moon" happening. Layers of hurt and grief build and take their toll as patient after patient progresses with the disease.

Being close to and identifying with patients or family members brings the health provider into more personal contact with them, which adds to the difficulty of mentally detaching from work. They may live through feelings of a personal loss again, as Dennis did for his father. They may, like Debbie, reflect on their own mortality and the meaning of life. Kim is stunned by the similarity in gestures, voice, and looks one patient had with her sister. The fact that this man is in the midst of a transsexual process to become a woman doesn't matter. Steve identifies with the white, upper-class, middle-aged, gay patients because they're like him and his friends. There but for the grace of God go I!

Realizing that people with AIDS have endless needs, caregivers often feel guilty if they can't respond to all of them. They feel remiss about leaving work at the end of their shifts or for vacations when there is always more to do. If patients with whom they've had long-term relationships die when the caregiver isn't at work, the health workers feel guilty. They also think they would feel irresponsible if they stopped contributing to AIDS care. Marlene feels that she'd be throwing away all of her hard-won expertise.

Depression, guilt, and feeling overwhelmed are parts of the range of emotions that the caregivers experience. There is also pain. It's a difficult realization that, regardless of the interventions, small improvements, intimacy with patients, comfort, and research, the person is still probably going to die. Laura used to think that physical therapy would save all the children. It doesn't.

There is pain from the so-called roller coaster effect of the cyclical nature of illness and improvement. On the way toward a currently fatal disease course, patients usually deteriorate greatly. Even if it takes years on a wellness–sickness cycle, this can be agonizing for the health care providers to witness since they connected through long-term relationships. It's also distressing to be on the receiving end of patients' anger and to be aware of societal attitudes of fear, stigma, and lack of dignity shown to people with AIDS. It's tormenting to be a bystander and watch unfulfilled lives end before dreams and goals are realized. Not being able to have closure with patients who die or move to another facility is also difficult for the care-givers. For Dennis, it's very unsatisfying if he can't emotionally wrap things up before the end.

Reactions to risk factors of transmission among health care professionals working with people with AIDS are surprisingly low key. Realizing the real-life risk of infection to themselves and the possible consequences of their own contamination, they clearly know that universal precautions are the most appropriate safety measures for all. Despite believing in the efficacy of these methods, they inconsistently use precautions and often carelessly gamble with their own safety. Needlestick injuries may seem very remote until one happens in their midst.

Caregivers perceive greater risk from tuberculosis, hepatitis, and other infections than from HIV. Because these other diseases are transmitted more easily, they hit closer to home than AIDS and become a real possibility. Everyone is aware of the risks and admits to at least a small fear of infection, but it doesn't paralyze their work efforts or stop them from giving the patients the benefit of human touch. Periodic testing for the HIV antibody provides a measure of reassurance, but caregivers are very aware that testing might be too little, too late. They feel a need to acknowledge, but not dwell on, the risk to themselves, to practice safe and careful procedures, and to concentrate on the needs of the patients in order to effectively fulfill their professional roles.

Where caregivers have at least a measure of fear of contamination, their families are more afraid of transmission to their loved ones. Kim says that if she got stuck with a dirty needle, she'd have to practice safe sex with her husband. Not only the caregiver is affected by this work. Finally, colleagues who don't work with people with AIDS show their anxiety by refusing to cover a vacation schedule for someone who works with these men, women, boys, and girls.

Caregivers also experience positive feelings. It's exciting to be involved in a continual flow of new interdisciplinary information and work in an environment of great need. It's also energizing to strive to improve the quality of someone's life. They need to decipher the care puzzle for each patient within the constraints of time and resources. Lastly, it's appealing to contribute to present and future directions of AIDS care and to educate patients, staff, and members of the community-at-large in prevention and health promotion.

Survival Skills: Dealing with the Meaning of Loss and Death

Although caregivers, such as Marlene, recognize the endless requirements for the patients, they fulfill their call to be in a helping role by working with extremely needy patients.

Health providers become more aware of the process of dying, especially during weeks when it becomes almost customary. Losses of dignity, independence, and dreams are evident as physical, and sometimes mental, deterioration occurs. Caregivers often have more trouble with these incremental losses than they do with the subsequent death. Kim believes that death is relatively easy after all of the other decline. In a climate where the highs are not very high, and the lows can be exceedingly low, caregivers can become off-balance. Elaine points out that rehabilitation professionals assist the patients to return home and resume activities of living. With AIDS care, she dolefully notes, "There is a death in there."

Occasionally, though, they feel a sense of relief when a patient's valiant struggle has ended. Even at those times, they can get sentimental when recalling patients and the anecdotes of their lives. Kim describes the scrapbook of patients that her group created, now fallen into disuse, which helps them lighten the experience and gain closure. A point is reached when humorous recollections no longer cause them to feel guilty, and they can enjoy the patients as people.

It's challenging to assist patients make peace with themselves. Caregivers help people deal with unresolved issues, regrets, and often the pain of dying too soon. As they do this, they also learn about themselves and find ways to cope with the situations they face. This allows them to more effectively help others manage overwhelming circum-stances.

Health providers who work with people with AIDS believe that it's their responsibility to find ways to contend with the inevitability of their patients' progressive decline and death, and they feel guilty that their methods are often inadequate. They help patients, families, and colleagues deal with so many issues, but they have a tendency to overlook their own needs for personal and professional survival. Protecting themselves from the devastation is a key survival technique, but in practice, the caregivers, as Marlene notes, get "sucked up." They try to set boundaries for their time and responsibilities by not working overtime or bringing work home, not talking about work off-the-job, and avoiding many wakes and funerals. Although they may attempt to guard themselves consistently, they also tend to ignore or overstep their own established guidelines. It appears that they know better intellectually, but emotionally they get caught up in the moment. They express a strong need to try to be everything to everyone.

Most caregivers choose not to attend funerals, wakes, or hospital memorial services. This avoidance is another way to separate personal and professional spheres and protect themselves. After going to only one funeral, Ann decided that one was enough. She said she'd be going all the time if she allowed herself. In the beginning, Laura felt a real need to go to the funerals to experience the reality of death. She, too, stopped that practice. When they spoke about other staff members who regularly attend funerals, they said that it wasn't healthy to make AIDS the central focus of their lives. It appears, though, that AIDS is, if not the central focus, highly meaningful and significant to them. More than just a job, this work seems to exact a commitment from its soldiers, which they willingly give. Even caregivers who feel burned out envision continuing their work with people with AIDS.

Grieving while still at work helps lessen the need to bring these emotions home. Caregivers think it's beneficial to share mutual feelings of sorrow and loss with their colleagues, who understand the depth and breadth of the experience. However, it's often difficult to share feelings and thoughts across the table of organization. Staff members may ventilate to a staff liaison, such as Debbie, the psychiatric nurse who facilitates a nurses' support group, but Debbie knows that it's not her role to discuss her feelings in that forum. Support meetings on particular units and wards are helpful to professionals who work in those areas, but people like Ann, who "float" throughout an organization, don't feel they belong in these sessions. They would be strangers baring their souls in someone else's home. The more sense of belonging a worker has, the greater communication takes place, and the less isolation is perceived by the caregiver.

Even loosely structured teamwork reinforces the concept that no one is alone and that no one person has to provide everything. Concerns and sentiments are shared and so is responsibility for care and outcome. Caregivers may understand the benefits, yet still not practice the team approach. Perhaps their strong inclination to fulfill helping roles is part of their problem.

A supportive, flexible work environment promotes professional freedom, decision making, and independence in scheduling one's time. Health workers who are able to change their activities when they're feeling overwhelmed enjoy their work more and feel less stress than employees in jobs where this flexibility doesn't exist. When tension mounts, caregivers tend to temporarily withdraw from patients or staff. Jessie is able to spend an afternoon researching at the library if emotions are building, and Steve can "waste fifteen minutes" walking or reading the sports page. These small breaks from the routine help sustain their mental health and their interest in the job. Rotating patients and duties among staff members also helps keep caregivers healthy so that they can continue their work. Educational or administrative responsibilities along with their clinical duties create diversions in the work day and form a protective shield so that providers don't interact with very ill, needy patients one hundred percent of the time.

Health workers also unwind by exercising, meditating, spending time with friends, families, and pets, and participating in other recreational and cultural activities. These important coping mechanisms help the caregivers separate from work, reduce stress, and have more balanced lives.

All Learning Great and Small: Personal and Professional Growth Issues

Moved and touched by patients, the caregivers are changed. They feel deeply about their patients' life circumstances and absorb their troubles. Confronting their personal demons of stereotyping and bigotry, like Mark did, they better understand the conflict they have with the values and beliefs they were taught. It's a time for examining their priorities and putting matters into perspective. Like Debbie, some caregivers now better understand their own vulnerability. As they continually manage their patients' problems, they're forced to look within themselves and at their own relationships. They're deciding who is important to them and who is just window-dressing and, therefore, expendable. Who is truly there for them and who do they choose to be there for? Life, they realize, is too short.

A firsthand view of dying helps them appreciate the quality of their lives and the well-being of their loves ones. Although they focus more clearly on their dreams and goals, they live in the present. Seeing the flame of so many young lives snuffed out emphasizes the need to fully experience their lives.

Observing human behavior, caregivers modify their perspectives. They notice the impact of ethnic, cultural, and religious differences upon their work, which in turn helps them understand the problems of minority and societal have-not groups. The stigma attached to AIDS causes people to maintain a conspiracy of silence, even at the risk of not getting needed benefits and support.

Their work provides lessons in anthropology and sociology as they get a bird's-eye view of what makes people tick. They need to motivate and care for people of various cultures, religious backgrounds, economic and educational levels. They become jaded about the goodness and responsibility of humans as they witness irresponsible behaviors of some HIV-infected people, such as unsafe sexual practices and subsequent pregnancies. On the other hand, health providers are surprised at the fortitude, resourcefulness, and courage of people with AIDS in the face of dying. Survival is a powerful motivator. As they absorb this information, they have the need to do something with it, to put it somewhere, but often are unsure of its place. Their professional outlook is altered, and they become increasingly introspective.

Even though life courses and class lines may differ between patient and caregiver, the professionals find things in common with their charges. It also amazes them that they have anything in common with sex workers, IV drug users, and prisoners.

Health providers are aware that the care models, by necessity, have changed, but they're uncertain of what the new model should be. Keeping patients healthy as long as possible is a goal. Improving physical and mental functioning is a goal. Regardless of the setting they work in, the health workers interviewed here don't accept throwing in the towel. They work to enhance the patient's welfare rather than accept the status quo. The shift in perspective of AIDS from a terminal to a chronic illness buoys their hopeful outlook and broadens their goals for the patients. People are living longer and managing health problems over many years.

Caregivers carefully assess their own skills and maturity. They get more in touch with the assets that they'd like to enhance, like compassion and thirst for learning. They also recognize their liabilities, such as anger and intolerance, which they'd prefer to change.

The opportunity to be on the cutting edge, a phrase used by most of the caregivers interviewed, motivates them to work with people with AIDS and adds to their self-worth and job satisfaction. They're excited by the contributions they make. New medications and more effective combinations of drugs continue to come on the scene. Care providers must continually keep up with the whirlpool of information and change the way they do their work.

Changing Challenges of Care: Finding Meaning in AIDS Care

How do the health care professionals find meaning in their jobs working with AIDS patients? Why do they remain in AIDS care? This gets at the heart of the matter. In trying to make sense of the meaning of their work, health care professionals working with people with AIDS have many emotions, thoughts, and concerns to sift through. From their stories, we know that they consider their work meaningful and a significant part of their lives. They also need to make sense of the experience. To accomplish this, they look at their relationships with patients, families, colleagues, systems, and people in their own lives. They express their feelings and name things in their world, such as the roller coaster effect.

Feeling like pioneers, an often repeated word, or veterans in their fields, gives them a sense of belonging and stature in the world. There are many subtle benefits of their jobs — opportunities to generously advocate for patients, promote positive changes for people, and foster growth.

Professionals agree that AIDS care certainly is challenging, but the word sometimes seems to be used euphemistically for "frustrating" and "problematic." There are advantages as well as pitfalls. They enjoy the search for answers and get excited by finding solutions. However, deciphering puzzles takes its toll when there are so many variables, such as insurance, housing, transportation, family support, dysfunctional behavior, and the disease itself. It's clear that challenges are not met without emotional cost to the caregivers.

The effectiveness continuum represents the best of times and the worst of times. Caregivers feel at their peak when resolving patients' problems, assisting them in resuming life activities, and providing resources to patients and clients who will follow-through on them. Teaching patients, families, and other colleagues to better understand AIDS and its consequences is high on their competency meter. In short, they feel best when they help patients thrive. On the other hand, they feel the least capable when they have little control over people and events. Occasionally, their own impatience, frustration, and anger gets the better of them. Sometimes, despite their efforts, they can't improve the behavior and attitude of patients and families. Patients resume substance abuse or high-risk sex. Families and friends don't always embrace the patients. Sometimes, the disease wins battles. Sometimes, it wins the war.

Work life on the roller coaster is stressful. The nature of AIDS is marked by steps forward and steps backward rather than by linear progression. There can be dramatic fluctuations in the physical and mental well-being of patients. Elaine and Debbie show us how these ups and downs affect their work and patient care. They also can wreak havoc with emotions.

Support from the family and friends of caregivers varies, but the more positive the support, the easier the job. Negative influences can undermine a person's choice of work, hamper "venting" about concerns, and result in feeling isolated.

Caregivers view AIDS as a medical illness, not a social disease. They don't condemn the patients. The disease simply is. No one deserves it.

The professionals interviewed here work with people who other caregivers shy away from. They are devoted to their patients and overextend themselves to the point of exhaustion. They jump into the fray, as Marlene notes, work longer hours than their shifts dictate, and strive to remove obstacles in patients' lives. They even donate their time on state-imposed furlough days. These care providers work to make a difference. They're proud of their work — and often exhausted.

Challenge, satisfaction, excitement, learning, and enjoyment seem to offset the sorrow, anguish, loss, and frustration inherent in working with people with AIDS. The health care professionals interviewed have been able to develop recuperative powers over time that allow them to stay in their jobs. Although they wonder about their future, no one has plans to leave their positions or stop doing AIDS care.

The professionals who are in the trenches doing this work are awesome! There is no other word for them. The fact that they keep doing what they do, and I get to help them, is a great thing.

Elaine, physical therapist

Chapter Thirteen

Help and Hope

From what we've learned in this book about caregivers who work with people with AIDS, it's possible to recommend guidelines to assist health professionals in their choice of clinical areas, maintain their well-being, support them in their work, and recruit, develop, and retain staff members. Certain key issues need to be addressed: staffing shortages, working conditions, and financial incentives to draw people to the helping professions and AIDS care. These problems are particularly noticeable in areas where differences among people are not as well accepted. There are inadequate numbers of health care professionals willing to provide essential care. In addition, many new graduates seem overwhelmed by the idea of working with people with AIDS.

The Organized Approach

Student and graduate health care professionals need to examine their own beliefs, feelings, and biases about people with AIDS so that the nature and character of the care they provide are not compromised. They can also gain information and understanding of lifestyles of people with AIDS, recognize homophobia in themselves and others, and work to unlearn prejudice. Clinical training manuals and organization-sponsored classes might be beneficial in aiding these efforts. Regularly scheduled seminars are recommended on issues such as role relationships, family dynamics, patient and family anger, and the sorrow, anguish, hostility, and pressures of caregivers.

Organizations should adopt policies to manage the stress and grief of AIDS care that contribute to burnout. Rotation of duties among staff members is shown to be helpful. Non-AIDS care can provide healthy down-time to revitalize employees in organizations where flexible scheduling is possible.

Ongoing caregiver support by consultants or liaisons, within or outside of the organization or unit, can help providers ventilate feelings, thoughts, and concerns and work through their issues. If the liaison also works with people with AIDS, care should be taken to provide support to this person as well. Opportunities for the professionals to debrief after a death may promote closure. Supportive, flexible environments that build strong morale of caregivers may reduce the incidence of burnout and provide incentives to work with people with AIDS.

Honest discussions about the risk of HIV transmission is essential on the community, educational program, and organizational levels. Ignorance appears to fuel the fear. There needs to be admission of the facts that risk does exist and universal precautions reduce, but don't eliminate, risk of HIV transmission. Educational presentations to large groups of student and graduate professionals are helpful to share facts and findings and correct misinformation, but smaller group discussions provide forums to acknowledge and confront fears. As long as a risk of transmission exists, there will be some degree of legitimate fear. Correcting inaccurate information and reinforcing consistent infection control procedures may reduce the worry. The anxiety of health care providers and their families and friends may reflect their perceived threat of AIDS, rather than the actual risk. Professionals who have worked through their fears are a good source for information and emotional support.

Academic curriculum development in professional programs should focus on improving communication skills, such as (a) acquiring social histories of patients, (b) educating patients and families about AIDS, (c) assessing what is being understood and the emotional reaction to the information, and (d) providing opportunities for patients to ask questions and share feelings and concerns. Training in these skills and in the emotional and psychological aspects of people with AIDS can be integrated into the curricula of professional health care schools and postgraduate programs, preparing new caregivers to face the demands of practice. The curriculum of tomorrow needs to be concerned with beliefs, values, and attitudes, as well as the factual knowledge of patient care.

Sufficient training in the area of AIDS may promote comfort, diminish fear, and assure competent care. There are many characteristics of AIDS that distinguish it from other clinical diseases and conditions — the fear of the disease and of people who have it; fluctuations in the course of the disease, which can undermine already arranged medical and social services; life-threatening illnesses that may involve many different systems of the body; a progressive course of the syndrome; and discrimination and breaches of confidentiality, which impact housing, employment, insurance, and personal support systems. An understanding of the distinctive characteristics of AIDS may help caregivers sensitively respond to the needs of patients.

Shifting Winds

The face of AIDS is changing. New treatments are giving people a second life. Once-emaciated young people, who looked decades older, are working out in gyms and returning to life. Some people who sold their possessions to pay for their treatments are now looking to return to work. Protease inhibitors are being hailed as miracle drugs, acting on the virus at different points in its reproductive cycle than do the other drugs like AZT, ddC, ddI, and 3TC. It would seem that a diagnosis of AIDS now heralds illness rather than death. Lest we become too complacent in our own preventive measures, we need to remember that as powerful as these medications are for many people, they're not effective for everyone. In addition, the expense and accessibility of the drugs keeps them out of reach for significant numbers of people in the United States and worldwide. Many poor people affected by AIDS contend with other social problems as well. Not everyone can manage the complicated medication regimen.

In the United States, we're seeing a decline of infections, but those numbers don't tell the whole story. Certain segments of our population, notably women and people of color, still show rising infection rates. HIV/AIDS is also spreading in other areas of the globe, such as eastern Europe and Asia.

Scientists are studying the factors that influence the rate at which the virus replicates and the impact on how long it takes for people to develop AIDS. They're researching defective genes that influence the progression of AIDS. The search continues for a preventive vaccine.

The focus is now shifting. It's a changing mindset of living with AIDS rather than dying with AIDS. It's easier to keep hope alive now, but it's a cautious optimism. Some medications are new, and clinical information is still being collected. Strategies may change. Long-term effectiveness cannot be determined. We may be climbing out of dark despair in certain parts of the world, but are we really on the twilight of this scourge?

As patients live longer, they will need more help, not less. Health professionals are having to develop new perspectives and models of care. Treatment goals still depend upon what body systems are affected. The nature of the disease necessitates continually changing goals and treatment regimens.

The Chord of Change

A particular theme strikes a chord that gently weaves together the past and present realities and casts hope on future directions. As the health care professionals interviewed here reflected upon their work with AIDS patients, they voiced an awareness of personal change. They were touched by the people in their care, and their perspectives on life and work were subsequently changed.

We may also be changed by their discoveries. Sharing their stories, we may have developed a better appreciation of the inherent difficulties of working with people with AIDS and a deeper respect for professionals who do the work. In addition, we may have been touched by the caring, concern, and commitment manifested by these health workers, sometimes in the face of hostility and abuse. I hope that we feel greater compassion for the people with AIDS, their families, friends, and caregivers in the face of this pandemic we call AIDS.

The work and growth continue.

I saw him be very ill, then improve, then "crump" again. I think this roller coaster ride with him was harder for me because I had known him over a longer period of time.

Elaine, physical therapist

10. Centers for Disease Control and Prevention. (1996). HIV/AIDS Surveillance Report, 8 (2), 7.

11. Centers for Disease Control and Prevention. (1996). HIV/AIDS Surveillance Report, 8 (2), 22.

12. Centers for Disease Control and Prevention. (1996). HIV/AIDS Surveillance Report, 8 (2), 13.

13. Centers for Disease Control and Prevention. (1996). HIV/AIDS Surveillance Report, 8 (2), 19.

14. "AIDS escalating; deaths exceed 100,000." *The Providence Journal-Bulletin,* p. A2, January 25, 1991.

15. Centers for Disease Control and Prevention. (1996). HIV/AIDS Surveillance Report, 8 (2), 21.

16. Centers for Disease Control and Prevention. (1996). HIV/AIDS Surveillance Report, 8 (2), 12.

17. Portis, K. "Breaking down barriers: HIV infection and communities of color." In J. B. Meisenhelder, and C. L. LaCharite (Eds.), *Comfort in Caring: Nursing the person with HIV infection,* (pp. 67-73). Boston, Mass.: Scott, Foresman and Company, 1989.

18. Simmonds, P., F. A. L. Lainson, R. Cuthbert, C. M. Steel, J. F. Peutherer, and C. A. Ludlam, "HIV antigen and antibody detection: Variable responses to infection in Edinburgh hemophiliac cohort." *British Medical Journal,* 296, 593-598. 1988.

19. Moss, A. R., P. Bacchetti, D. Osmond, W. Krampf, R. E. Chaisson, D. Stites, J. Wilber, J. P. Allain, and J. Carlson, "Seropositivity for HIV and the development of AIDS or AIDS-related conditions: Three-year follow-up of the San Francisco General Hospital cohort." *British Medical Journal,* 296, 745-750. 1988.

20.   Meisenhelder, J. B. "Overcoming the fear." In J. B.
       Meisenhelder, and C. L. LaCharite (Eds.), *Comfort
       in Caring: Nursing the person with HIV infection,*
       (pp. 3-11). Boston, Mass.: Scott, Foresman and
       Company, 1989.

21.   Friedland, G. H., and R. S. Klein, "Transmission of
       the human immunodeficiency virus." 317 (18),
       1125-1135. *New England Journal of Medicine,*
       1987.

22.   Centers for Disease Control. "Update: Human
       immunodeficiency virus infections in health care
       workers exposed to blood of infected patients."
       Morbidity and Mortality Weekly Report, 36 (19),
       285-287, 1987.

23.   Van der Graaf, M., and R. J. A. Diepersloot,
       "Transmission of human immunodeficiency virus
       (HIV/HTLV-III/LAV): A review." *Infection,* 14 (5),
       203-211. 1986.

24.   Friedland, G. H., and R. S. Klein, "Transmission of
       the human immunodeficiency virus." 317 (18),
       1125-1135. *New England Journal of Medicine,*
       1987.
       Sande, M. A. "Transmission of AIDS: The case
       against casual contagion." *New England Journal of
       Medicine,* 314 (6), 380-382. 1986.

25.   Hoff, L. A. *People in Crises: Understanding and
       helping* (3rd ed.). Reading, Mass.: Addison-Wesley
       Publishing Company, Inc., 1989.

26.   Feinblum, S. "Pinning down the psychosocial
       dimensions of AIDS." *Nursing and Health Care,* 7
       (5), 255-257. 1987.

About the Author

Director of Adaptive Health Associates, Inc., in Rhode Island, Meredith E. Drench, PhD, PT is a speaker, consultant, and educator, specializing in behavior and health care. Working with sensitive issues in the workplace and community, she values and emphasizes communication, ethical empowerment, and collaboration, as she helps people become more effective in their lives.

Dr. Drench's work with AIDS/HIV has taken her to Eastern and Western Europe and throughout the United States. She has presented her research at the National Institute of Hematology in Budapest, the International Conference on AIDS, the Annual Conference of the American Physical Therapy Association (APTA), and the Annual Research Symposium of Rhode Island's Chapter of APTA.

Meredith has published articles in health care and behavior and has been a contributing author to the books *Issues in HIV Rehabilitation; Nursing Focus: Psychological Adaptation to Disability and Chronic Illness;* and *Perspectives: Human Sexuality.*

To order additional copies of

Red Ribbons Are Not Enough

Book: $14.95   Shipping/Handling $3.50

Contact: ***BookPartners, Inc.***
P.O. Box 922, Wilsonville, OR 97070
Fax: 503-682-8684
Phone 503-682-9821
Phone: 1-800-895-7323